THE AMERICAN
DIABETES ASSOCIATION

# GUIDE
# TO HERBS &
# NUTRITIONAL
# SUPPLEMENTS

What You Need to Know from
## Aloe to Zinc

## LAURA SHANE-MCWHORTER
### PharmD, BCPS, FASCP, BC-ADM, CDE

*Contributing Writer,* Kate Ruder; *Director, Book Publishing,* Robert Anthony; *Managing Editor, Book Publishing,* Abe Ogden; *Production Manager,* Melissa Sprott; *Cover Design,* Jody Billert; *Printer,* Data Reproductions Corporation.

Printed in the United States of America
1 3 5 7 9 10 8 6 4 2

The suggestions and information contained in this publication are generally consistent with the *Clinical Practice Recommendations* and other policies of the American Diabetes Association, but they do not represent the policy or position of the Association or any of its boards or committees. Reasonable steps have been taken to ensure the accuracy of the information presented. However, the American Diabetes Association cannot ensure the safety or efficacy of any product or service described in this publication. Individuals are advised to consult a physician or other appropriate health care professional before undertaking any diet or exercise program or taking any medication referred to in this publication. Professionals must use and apply their own professional judgment, experience, and training and should not rely solely on the information contained in this publication before prescribing any diet, exercise, or medication. The American Diabetes Association—its officers, directors, employees, volunteers, and members—assumes no responsibility or liability for personal or other injury, loss, or damage that may result from the suggestions or information in this publication.

⊚ The paper in this publication meets the requirements of the ANSI Standard Z39.48-1992 (permanence of paper).

ADA titles may be purchased for business or promotional use or for special sales. To purchase more than 50 copies of this book at a discount, or for custom editions of this book with your logo, contact the American Diabetes Association at the address below, at booksales@diabetes.org, or by calling 703-299-2046.

American Diabetes Association
1701 North Beauregard Street
Alexandria, Virginia 22311

DOI: 10.2337/9781580403184

**Library of Congress Cataloging-in-Publication Data**

Shane-McWhorter, Laura.
 The American Diabetes Association guide to herbs and nutritional supplements : what you need to know from aloe to zinc / Laura Shane-McWhorter.
   p. cm.
 Includes bibliographical references and index.
 ISBN 978-1-58040-318-4 (alk. paper)
 1. Diabetes--Alternative treatment. 2. Diabetes--Diet therapy. 3. Dietary supplement. 4. Herbs--Therapeutic use. I. American Diabetes Association. II. Title. III. Title: Guide to herbs and nutritional supplements.
 RC661.A47S528 2009
 616.4'6206--dc22
                    2009033623

# CONTENTS

# PREFACE

As a pharmacist for more than twenty years, I have worked with hundreds of people who want to use dietary supplements to better treat their diabetes. Some people view supplements as healthier alternatives to "harsh" prescription medications. Others take dietary supplements in addition to prescribed medications to treat their blood glucose or complications of diabetes. What all these patients need is guidance on the benefits and cautions of using these substances.

Two of my patients with diabetes who have used dietary supplements (their names and some details have been changed) illustrate this need.

One patient was a middle-aged woman named Jackie, who had just been diagnosed with type 2 diabetes. She had already been taking medications for her high blood pressure and depression. Jackie's doctor recommended that she check her blood glucose regularly, take a new prescription diabetes medication, and lose 20 pounds by eating well and exercising more regularly.

Jackie decided that there must be a "better way," so she made a trip to her local vitamin store to ask about products that she could use instead of prescription medications. At the vitamin store, an eager, pleasant employee told Jackie that she should start taking a variety of products such as ginseng, bitter melon, fenugreek, chromium, and vanadium. When Jackie asked whether she should be aware of any side effects or drug interactions, the well-meaning store clerk told her that dietary supplements are "natural" and do not have any side effects or drug interactions. Jackie was so encouraged that she stopped taking her prescription medications and bought only "natural" products for her high blood pressure, depression, and newly diagnosed diabetes.

After a few weeks, Jackie returned to her doctor because she was not feeling well, and she thought that she might have a bladder infection. Her doctor asked whether she was taking her newly prescribed diabetes medication, as well as her medications for high blood pressure and depression. Jackie explained that she was taking only "natural" products. Her doctor then informed her that her blood glucose and blood pressure were sky high and that she did indeed have a bladder infection.

Another patient I remember was David—a lean, well-educated retired professor of anthropology. David's physician had referred David to me to discuss his dietary supplement use. He had recently been diagnosed with diabetes, and he had made many lifestyle changes in order to treat his diabetes. He gave up eating meats of any sort and became a strict vegetarian. He started walking—then running—about 2 miles daily. He also purchased many dietary supplements. When he showed me his supplements (about 17 different bottles) I asked him why he was taking each of the products. Some were to increase energy, some were for high blood pressure, some were for high cholesterol, and some were for diabetes. He had started these products because he felt that a natural approach would be best to treat his medical conditions. After scrutinizing the bottles and ingredients, I noted that many of the products had some of the same ingredients, and several of the products had very high doses of vitamins. Furthermore, although David had indeed lost about 10% of his body weight, and his blood pressure, cholesterol, and blood glucose levels had decreased somewhat, they were still higher than target goals. My advice was to consolidate some of the different products and then to reinstate his prescription medications.

*     *     *     *     *

Where should Jackie and David have turned for information on taking dietary supplements? There isn't an easy answer. Some patients have a strong desire to self-treat a disease such as diabetes with dietary supplements. This desire may come from the emotional component of wellness and healing and the widely held belief that dietary supplements are "natural" and can thus cause no harm.

This book is intended to help others like Jackie and David find more information about commonly used dietary supplements for diabetes and its related conditions. This book *does not* recommend specific supplements or brands. Instead, it gives general information on the safety and efficacy of some commonly used supplements. It also provides specific information about how supplements work, possible side effects and drug interactions, and suggestions as to what patients should look for if they decide to use a particular product. Patients should always talk with their health care providers about any dietary supplements they are planning to take.

# ACKNOWLEDGMENTS

I would like to thank my family, friends, and administrative personnel, who have provided much encouragement, support, and counsel during my work on this book. Specifically, I would like to thank my husband, Jerry, as well as my children, Chris, Sandy, Randy, and David, and my grandson, Cody. I would like to give a special thank-you to my friend Dick for his invaluable technical support.

This book would not be possible without the vision that Victor Van Beuren had about writing a consumer guide. I would also like to acknowledge Kate Ruder for her sage advice and expertise in writing consumer guides in the area of diabetes.

# PART I
## INTRODUCTION

You want to live healthy and well with your diabetes. You try to visit your health care provider regularly, take your prescribed medications, eat a balanced diet, and exercise regularly. Yet, there is one aspect of your health that may not be addressed in your regular medical visits, but you may still have questions about—taking dietary supplements.

Today, more and more people use dietary supplements. It's a multibillion-dollar-a-year industry. And studies show that people with diabetes are more likely to use supplements than people without diabetes. The National Health Interview Survey found that 22 percent of people with diabetes used some type of herbal therapy, while another study found that 31 percent used dietary supplements. Certain ethnic groups, such as Hispanics, Native Americans, Asians, and African Americans are also more likely to use dietary supplements.

If you're one of the many people taking dietary supplements, you're probably concerned about doing the right thing for your body. People with diabetes who use complementary and alternative medicines, such as supplements, tend to have healthy habits. One study found that they're more likely to visit their primary care providers and get their flu shots. However, finding reliable information about the benefits and safety of these products is difficult. There are hundreds of dietary supplements—each purporting their own health benefits. You've probably browsed the vitamin aisle at the pharmacy or a health food store. Maybe you felt overwhelmed so you didn't purchase anything, or you just grabbed a supplement marketed for people with diabetes. In either case, you probably had unanswered questions about the safety and efficacy of these products.

## How to Use This Book

So, what's a discerning consumer to do? First, read this book. It's intended to give you enough information about dietary supplements to have an educated discussion with your health care provider. You should always consult your health care provider when making any change to your medication regimen, and taking a dietary supplement is no exception.

This section, Part I, discusses what dietary supplements are, why you should exercise caution when taking supplements, and how to talk to your health care provider. It also describes how dietary supplements are regulated and how to shop wisely for these products.

Part II summarizes 40 dietary supplements commonly used to treat diabetes and its complications. This is not a comprehensive directory of all the dietary supplements used to treat diabetes—just a snapshot of the most well-known products. The supplements are listed in alphabetical order so that you can easily look up a product in which you're interested or considering taking. Each summary includes details on the supplement's origin, general information about how the product is thought to work, potential side effects and drug interactions, and relevant scientific studies.

Part III summarizes the information from Part II into a quick-reference table, making it easier to locate and read a brief summary of a particular supplement. While this table makes it convenient to identify a supplement quickly, it is recommended that you also read the full entry for any supplement in which you are interested.

## TYPES OF DIETARY SUPPLEMENTS

Dietary supplements include everything from vitamins and minerals to herbs such as cinnamon and St. John's wort. Hundreds of plant species have been used to treat diabetes throughout the ages. Indeed, the widely prescribed drug metformin belongs to a class of drugs that is related to the plant French lilac, or goat's rue. Dietary supplements also come in a number of forms including tablets, capsules, powders, softgels, gelcaps, and liquids. And they are sold from a number of retailers including pharmacies, grocery stores, vitamin and health food stores, websites, and mail-order catalogs.

The main types of dietary supplements this book will cover include:

- Botanicals (derived from plants and possibly including herbs)
- Vitamins
- Minerals
- Fatty Acids
- Other Dietary Supplements

## REASONS FOR CAUTION: SIDE EFFECTS AND DRUG INTERACTIONS

Dietary supplements may seem safe or mild because they're natural. Many think that something natural couldn't hurt them. Yet, serious side effects and drug interactions can occur when taking dietary supplements. For example, supplements such as aloe vera, fenugreek, and vanadium may cause excessive bleeding during surgery or interact with anesthetics. Other supplements may interfere with prescription medications. For instance, ginseng may be used to treat diabetes, but may interfere with the drug warfarin's ability to prevent blood clotting. St. John's wort, which people often take for depression, can interact with antidepressants, as well as many other prescription medications. In Part II, you'll find more examples of side effects and drug interactions for individual supplements.

Your health care provider is the best resource for assessing the risks and benefits of taking a dietary supplement. He or she should know the potential side effects of supplements—and the risk for interactions with your other medications.

## Talking to Your Health Care Provider

Despite the risks, people generally don't tell their health care providers that they take dietary supplements. A recent analysis found that 69% of patients who use prescription medications and dietary supplements do not talk about supplements with their health care providers. Certain ethnic groups, such as Hispanics, are less likely than others to tell their health care providers that they take supplements.

Patients may not consider these products "drugs," or they may just forget to mention them during their doctor's visits. Patients may also think their health care providers will disapprove of their choices. Not disclosing supplement use can present dangerous circumstances. For example, a patient may experience a side effect of a dietary supplement that the provider may then attribute to another medication.

Your pharmacist, doctor, or diabetes educator is the most reliable source for information about the safety and efficacy of dietary supplements. Pharmacists are the most accessible of all health care providers. While retailers in health food stores may seem knowledgeable, they probably don't have the medical background or familiarity with your personal health to recommend products. The same is true for retailers on the Internet.

Following are some tips for talking with your doctor, pharmacist or diabetes educator:

- Always tell your doctor about any supplements you're taking, including multivitamins. List them as medications in your written records.

- Tell your doctor why you are taking that supplement.

- Don't wait for your doctor to ask you about your supplement use. Many health care providers forget to ask about these products.

- Conversely, tell your doctor if you intend to stop or have already stopped taking a supplement.

- If you're planning to take a new supplement, ask whether it has any side effects or interactions with other medications or supplements, or whether it may interact with another one of your medical conditions.

- Ask how the supplement might affect your health—including your blood glucose, blood pressure, cholesterol, or other medical conditions.

- Your doctor might recommend that you take one product at a time to evaluate how your body reacts. He or she may recommend that you monitor your blood glucose more closely when you start taking a new supplement.

- Make a list of the supplements you take before your appointment, or put the bottles in a bag and bring them with you. Also list in what dose, how often, and for how long you've been taking the supplement.

- Never stop taking your traditional diabetes medications without telling your health care provider.

- Continue to be forthright about the supplements you're taking, even if your doctor has discouraged their use.

---

## WHERE TO RESEARCH YOUR DIETARY SUPPLEMENTS ONLINE

If your doctor is unsure about possible side effects or drug interactions, you may want to research information to share with your doctor. The following websites are good places to start:

http://www.nlm.nih.gov/medlineplus/dietarysupplements.html#cat42

U.S. National Library of Medicine and National Institutes of Health, "Medline Plus: Dietary Supplements"

http://ods.od.nih.gov/factsheets/DietarySupplements.asp

National Institutes of Health Office of Dietary Supplements, "Dietary Supplements: Background Information"

http://nccam.nih.gov/health/bottle

National Institutes of Health National Center for Complementary and Alternative Medicine, "Get the Facts: What's in the Bottle? An Introduction to Dietary Supplements"

http://dietarysupplements.nlm.nih.gov/dietary

National Institutes of Health and U.S. National Library of Medicine Dietary Supplements Labels Database

---

## REGULATION OF DIETARY SUPPLEMENTS

If you believe the U.S. Food and Drug Administration (FDA) approves dietary supplements, you are not alone. A 2002 poll showed that 58 percent of Americans believe that government agencies, such as the FDA, must approve herbal products before they can be sold to the public.

However, dietary supplements *do not* need FDA approval.

Under legislation passed in 1994, called the Dietary Supplement Health and Education Act, supplements are considered foods, not drugs. Therefore, supplements do not have to undergo the same stringent approval process as drugs. Supplement manufacturers do not have to prove the safety, quality, or efficacy of their products before they arrive on shelves.

This reclassification has resulted in serious consequences. Sometimes contaminants or substitutes have been found in products. For instance, some diabetes products have been contaminated with lead, and other products touted as being "herbal" have contained prescription drugs.

How do these dangerous lapses occur? Because of the Dietary Supplement Health and Education Act, the FDA does not routinely analyze the contents of dietary supplements for their safety or efficacy. The manufacturer—not the government—is responsible for ensuring that the label is accurate and the ingredients are safe. Indeed, the FDA would have to prove that a supplement were unsafe in order to be allowed to remove it from the market.

## LABELS AND CONTENTS

Although limited in its oversight, the FDA requires manufacturers of dietary supplements to follow certain guidelines when describing their products. For example, manufacturers of dietary supplements can make claims regarding the ability to maintain "structure and function" of the body, but cannot make claims regarding diagnosis, treatment, cure, or prevention of disease. The label must include the following statement: "This statement has not been evaluated by the Food and Drug Administration (FDA). This product is not intended to diagnose, treat, cure, or prevent any disease." The manufacturer must notify the FDA within 30 days after a product is on the market if it bears such a label.

The FDA also bans implied, as well as expressed, disease treatment claims. In other words, claims made by a manufacturer that a buyer could misconstrue as indicating treatment or prevention of a disease are no longer allowed. In new regulations, a product may make health maintenance claims but not disease treatment claims (i.e., "maintains a healthy prostate" is allowed, but "treats benign prostatic hyperplasia" is not).

The FDA requires that supplement labels (see Figure 1) contain certain information, so look for these details when you shop for products.

- Name of the product

- Name and address of the manufacturer

- Complete list of ingredients, including a "Supplement Facts" panel, which identifies each ingredient in the product. If an ingredient is not listed on the "Supplement Facts" panel, it must be listed in the "other ingredients" statement below the panel.

- Directions for use

- Net quantity of the contents

Despite these requirements, the labels of dietary supplements can be confusing and misleading. A study of more than 800 bottles of popular herbs sold in retail stores found that over

| Supplement Facts | | |
|---|---|---|
| Serving Size: 1 capsule | | |
| Servings Per Container: 90 | | |
| | Amount per serving | %DV |
| Alpha-Lipoic Acid | 100 mg | * |
| * Daily Value not established. | | |

FIGURE 1.
Sample Supplement Label

half the products were inconsistent in reporting benchmark ingredients and recommended daily doses.

In addition, the actual contents of products may not be reflected in the packaging. A study of the popular botanical Echinacea, which is taken to relieve cold symptoms, found numerous discrepancies in the ingredients listed on products. Ten percent of "Echinacea" products contained no measurable Echinacea.

# INDEPENDENT TESTING
# ORGANIZATIONS

Luckily, a handful of independent organizations test the accuracy of the labels and contents of dietary supplements. They offer "seals of approval" that you may want to look for when shopping for supplements. However, keep in mind that these organizations do not test the efficacy of products.

## U.S. Pharmacopeia (USP) Dietary Supplement Verification Program

The "USP-verified mark" on the label indicates the label product ingredients are accurate and that the product is pure, will dissolve properly, and has been manufactured using good manufacturing practices. The USP website also lists manufacturers that have undergone the evaluation process (*www.usp.org*).

## NSF International

Formerly known as National Sanitation Foundation, NSF International verifies the accuracy of supplement labels and contents, checks for purity and contaminants, and audits the manufacturing process for good manufacturing practice compliance (*www.nsf.org*).

### Consumer Lab

Consumer Lab tests supplements for the accuracy and purity of their ingredients (*www.consumerlab.com*).

### The Consumers Union

The Consumers Union also tests certain products and reports findings in its publication, *Consumer Reports* (*www.consumerreports.com*; subscription required for some content).

### The Natural Products Association

The Natural Products Association has launched a good manufacturing practice program (*www.naturalproductsassoc.org*).

## Sizing Up the Product and Manufacturer

It's best to use a dietary supplement that comes in a pure, standardized form. You can check the purity of a product by consulting the United States Pharmacopoeia (www.usp.org). You'll also want to purchase products from large, nationally known companies. These companies are more likely to incorporate good manufacturing practices and stringent quality assurance.

If you have questions about a product, you may want to contact the manufacturer directly. The manufacturer should be able to answer the following questions:

- Has your product been evaluated in scientific studies that have been published in reputable medical journals? If so, are you willing to share these studies? Or, is most of the product information the result of testimonials by people with diabetes who have used the product?

- Can you explain how the product works? Do you have scientific studies that verify the mechanism of action?

- Does your company conduct a chemical analysis of the active and inactive ingredients to verify that the product contains what it says on the label?

- Does the product break down and dissolve appropriately in the stomach?

- Does your company specify specific storage or stability instructions, such as what temperature to store the product, whether light may affect the product, or whether it should be stored in a dark place? Do you list an expiration date for the shelf life of the product?

- Do you specify any side effects or possible interactions with other supplements or prescription drugs or disease states? Do you specify which patients should not use the product?

Even when armed with these questions and the best intentions, consumers may find it difficult to evaluate the safety and efficacy of products. Unfortunately, many of the scientific studies done on dietary supplements are unreliable. For example, studies may include only small numbers of patients. Some scientists never examine the actual contents of the studied products, so their results could be unintentionally skewed. For these reasons and others, the Natural Standard, an independent group of scientists who evaluate complementary and alternative medicines, has given most dietary supplements for diabetes a grade "B" or lower in terms of efficacy.

In Part II, you'll find summaries of the best studies done on each individual supplement, as well as tips for evaluating the results. Keep in mind that some supplements have been more rigorously studied than others. It's always best to talk with you health care provider about questions regarding the efficacy and safety of a product, rather than trying to troubleshoot on your own.

# How Much Should You Take?

The National Academy of Sciences provides information on reference daily intake (RDI) for many—but not all—vitamins and minerals. Most other dietary supplements, such as herbs, do not have recommended daily allowances. In fact, the appropriate doses of many dietary supplements are unknown. In Part II, you'll find the available information on recommended doses for individual supplements.

Some dietary supplements are sold in "packs" to people with diabetes. These packs may contain a handful of supplements marketed for improving diabetes. These products can make it difficult for patients to evaluate their responses to individual supplements. Instead of taking supplements together as they are packaged, take only one supplement at a time to determine your body's response when beginning new products. However, if you wish to take a "pack," then make sure you obtain it from a reputable manufacturer and discuss this with your doctor. Then the doctor may assess the impact on the control of your diabetes or other medical conditions.

# Tips from the FDA

Because manufacturers may use deceptive marketing tactics to promote their products, the FDA has put together a number of helpful resources for evaluating products.

## "How to Spot Health Fraud"

Web article available at *www.fda.gov*

This website warns against a single product that the manufacturers claim benefits a variety of unrelated diseases (i.e., difficulties ranging from menstrual problems to asthma to rheumatic complaints). It also suggests buyers be wary of evidence of benefit based on personal testimonials, claims of unusually rapid benefit, or use of meaningless phrases that may sound scientifically impressive to lay consumers but do not actually describe a beneficial medicinal effect.

## "Tips for the Savvy Supplement User"

Web article available at *www.cfsan.fda.gov*

Includes basic points to consider, such as talking with a health care provider before using a supplement and broaching the issue that some supplements may interact with prescription or over-the-counter medicines or have untoward effects during surgery. It also provides information on how to report adverse effects of dietary supplements. Furthermore, it provides tips on searching the Internet for information on supplements, including pointers on how to find out who operates a product website, the purpose of the site, the information sources and references, and whether the information is current.

## "Tips for Older Dietary Supplement Users"

Web article available at *www.cfsan.fda.gov*

Discusses potential risks, such as the danger of substitution of dietary supplements for conventional medications or consuming more than recommended amounts. It also advocates discussion of dietary supplement use with a health care provider. It provides a checklist of important considerations such as issues with side effects, drug interactions, and possible discontinuation before scheduled surgery.

## Contacting the FDA to report an issue

The FDA encourages patients and their health care providers to report any adverse effects related to dietary supplements through the FDA's MedWatch online at *www.fda.gov/safety/medwatch/default.htm* or by calling 1-800-FDA-1088.

# A Note on Clinical Studies

There is a lot of perplexing information regarding supplement products. When deciding whether or not to use a particular supplement, it is important for you as a consumer to understand information about different clinical studies, especially since the media may not always accurately represent the information from studies. Many times, the reporting on clinical studies leaves out important details or fails to mention how the study was conducted. This means that results from poorly designed studies are sometimes given more credence than they deserve, and results from well-run trials may be cherry-picked for the most sensational tidbits.

In this book, each supplement or herb has information about different studies regarding the type of scientific evaluations that have been published. Thus, to better understand the significance of these studies, knowing some important definitions and terms is essential.

## What are the characteristics of a good clinical study?

A clinical study is simply an experiment where a researcher tests whether a specific product (such as a medication, herb, or supplement) or a type of intervention (such as a special diet or a certain type of exercise) will work to achieve a certain endpoint. An "endpoint" is simply an event or outcome that has been defined and that a clinical study will evaluate. For instance, an endpoint may be losing a certain amount of weight, or improving a certain disease, symptom, or a laboratory value such as blood glucose or cholesterol.

Not all studies are equal, however, and it is important to understand the characteristics of a good clinical study. The most important aspect of a clinical study is how it is set up—this is called the "study design." The study design is critical in determining whether the published results are reliable enough to help you decide whether a product is worth taking. Some of the characteristics of a good study include the following:

- It is "randomized, double-blind, and placebo-controlled"
- It includes a large number of patients
- It has well-defined events or endpoints
- It has been evaluated mathematically by appropriate statistical analysis

What do all of these terms mean? The following is an explanation of important terms related to clinical studies.

*Randomization*: This method assigns an individual or patient to a particular study group or intervention based on chance. This decreases the possibility of some sort of "bias" or result that favors a particular treatment.

*Double blind*: This means that the medication, supplement, or intervention being used in the study is hidden from both the patient and the researcher. In other words, neither the patient nor the researcher knows what the patient is taking (no one knows whether the patient is taking the medication, or supplement, or a "dummy pill") and both the researcher and the patient are "blind" to what is being used. The purpose of a "double-blind" design is to decrease the possibility of "bias," since knowing what treatment is being used may influence either party.

*Placebo*: This is an inactive or "dummy pill" or treatment that looks and tastes and smells like the real product. The purpose of a placebo group is to compare the effectiveness of the active treatment or real medication, supplement, or herb against something that has no treatment value (the placebo).

*Endpoint*: An endpoint is an event that has been pre-defined and is being measured in the clinical study. For instance, examples of an "endpoint" would be a change in A1C (to see whether or not there is diabetes improvement), a change in pain scores (to determine improvement in pain due to neuropathy), or a change in laboratory values such as LDL cholesterol (the "bad" type of cholesterol).

An excellent "endpoint" is one that measures an effect on mortality (death) or on morbidity (a disease outcome such as heart attack or stroke; or on adverse occurrence such as blindness, nerve damage or amputations, or kidney failure). A good study that shows decreases in mortality and morbidity has usually been conducted for a long period of time (for years) and has a sufficiently large number of patients to demonstrate a benefit.

*Open-label*: In an open-label study, both the researcher and the patient know what is being taken. This type of study design introduces "bias," possibly because of the power of suggestion. Hence, an "open-label" study is not optimal.

*Run-in*: A run-in is a phase or period where no treatment is being given, often at the beginning of a study. This is sometimes done to provide some sort of baseline observation or to try to eliminate persons who may not cooperate. For instance, if a participant does not show up for important pre-study meetings or treatments, they probably will not comply with the treatments being studied (such as sticking to a diet).

*Washout*: This is the period of time needed for a drug or herb or other treatment to be eliminated from the body. Some times a "run-in" may be called a "washout" to allow enough time for the drug or herb to be cleared out from the body. An adequate "washout" becomes important when a participant is being changed to a different treatment during the study.

*Cross-over*: In a cross-over study, patients are given a certain medication, supplement, or herb for a period of time, and then the researchers might change them ("cross-over") to a different medication or supplement. A well-run cross-over study will also include a washout, since this allows time for the first treatment to be cleared from the body. If patients are "crossed-over" directly (without a "washout"), then the first medication or supplement may still be in the body, and the results may be falsely influenced by the treatment that is still in the body.

*"Statistically significant" or "significant results"*: These are mathematically analyzed results that are meaningful. For instance, a supplement may decrease blood glucose, but the results may not be statistically significant. Thus, even though the product has shown some benefit, the results are not strong enough or "significant" enough to justify taking the product. The opposite is also true—although sometimes the results are statistically significant, they are not enough to get a patient to his or her desired goals. For instance, a product may decrease fasting glucose "significantly" from 250 to 200 mg/dl, but the results are not at the desired goal of 70–130 mg/dl.

*Participants*: When determining the merit of a study or trial, it is also important to consider the participants. This information is almost never reported in major media coverage of trials, but can usually be found in the original published reports or with a little digging on the Internet. Factors to consider include:

- Who were the patients that participated? Were they healthy or did they actually have the disease that was being studied? A study focused on a blood glucose treatment but filled with non-diabetes participants would be less useful than the same study using people with diabetes.

- What were the characteristics of the patients at the start of the clinical trial? The patients in each group should have similar characteristics (for instance, age, health status, gender, or ethnicity) at the beginning of a well-run clinical trial. Differences in characteristics at the start could potentially affect the results, making the findings potentially less trustworthy.

- How many patients dropped out? If there is a difference between the study groups due to dropouts, then perhaps there could be a problem. For instance, if many people dropped out of the treatment group but the results are very favorable in that group, then the results may be suspicious because the sample size is smaller and people who responded negatively may not be represented in the final findings.

While there are many more terms, methods, and definitions associated with clinical studies, this list should cover most of what is discussed in the following text. Most important is that you remain vigilant as a consumer of medications and supplements. When you learn the results of a study, you should also learn how the study was conducted before making a decision. Search out literature on clinical trials and studies, and discuss studies with your doctor or pharmacist.

# PART II
## SUPPLEMENTS

# ALOE
## *Aloe vera*

This succulent, green tropical plant has been used in medicine for thousands of years. Aloe is pictured on the walls of ancient Egyptian temples and discussed for its medicinal properties in the Egyptian Book of Remedies from the 16th century. Derived from the Arabic *alloeh*, the name means "bitter and shiny substance." The plant thrives in warm climates such as the Mediterranean and Caribbean, as well as areas of Africa and North and South America. Aloe is just one of 400 species of aloe plants.

## USES

Patients are probably most familiar with aloe gel to treat sunburns, skin abrasions, and dry skin. However, aloe gel, which comes from the plant's leaves, is also the most common form used to treat diabetes. Aloe is popular among Hispanic patients and is known as *sábila*.

Aloe is taken by mouth to treat type 2 diabetes. It is found in many formulations such as beverage mixtures or tablets. The gel's active ingredients include polysaccharides and glycoprotein. They are thought to stimulate the body's ability to transport excess glucose from the blood into cells and tissues where it is needed. Some scientists suspect that the high fiber content of the gel itself may promote the body to use glucose more effectively. Nonetheless, aloe's effect on blood glucose has not been confirmed in large, rigorous, long-term studies.

Aloe latex is another form of aloe. It has a laxative effect and can be taken as a juice or dried and taken as a tablet. It is not used to treat diabetes.

## DOSE

There is no recommended dose, since necessary dose-finding studies have not been conducted.

## STUDIES

Three small studies have indicated that aloe may decrease blood glucose. It may also decrease triglycerides but not total cholesterol.

- A study of five patients with type 2 diabetes who took one-half teaspoon of aloe sap twice daily found that average blood glucose decreased. But the study was very small and did not include control subjects (i.e., patients who did not take aloe).

- A small study of 40 patients with type 2 diabetes who took one tablespoon of aloe gel or a placebo ("dummy gel") twice a day for 6 weeks found that fasting blood glucose decreased significantly in the aloe group. Triglyceride levels also decreased, but not overall cholesterol.

- In another small study of 40 patients with type 2 diabetes, scientists found that adding one tablespoon of aloe gel to the diabetes medication glyburide (a sulfonylurea) twice a day for 6 weeks significantly decreased fasting blood glucose. Triglyceride levels also decreased, but not overall cholesterol.

# Side Effects and Drug Interactions

There are many theoretical adverse effects of aloe. Patients should be cautious about low blood glucose when taking aloe in addition to diabetes medications such as insulin, sulfonylureas, and others.

In addition, patients should be cautious that an aloe product could be inadvertently contaminated with other parts of the plant that cause a laxative effect. For example, an ingredient found in aloe called anthraquinones was once included in over-the-counter laxatives. The FDA had concerns about fluid and electrolyte loss and had requested that manufacturers conduct further safety studies. Due to the excessive costs necessary to conduct these tests, manufacturers chose not to do the tests, and aloe is no longer allowed in nonprescription laxatives.

There are anecdotal reports of liver and kidney problems with high doses of aloe. Aloe should not be used by pregnant or breastfeeding women. There is concern that use during pregnancy may result in miscarriage and that some toxic substances may pass to the infant in breast milk.

There is the potential for prolonged bleeding when aloe is used with the anesthetic sevoflurane during surgery. Thus, aloe use should be stopped two weeks before surgery. Aloe should not be used with drugs that deplete potassium, such as certain diuretics. It should not be taken with the heart medication digoxin, since low potassium may result in dangerously high concentrations of digoxin.

# ALPHA-LIPOIC ACID

Alpha-lipoic acid is a vitamin-like substance called an anti-oxidant—a substance that protects cells from the damaging effects of oxidative stress. Scientists theorize that oxidative stress can lead to diseases such as cancer, heart disease, and diabetes. Alpha-lipoic acid is produced in the liver. In addition, alpha-lipoic acid is found in foods like broccoli, spinach, potatoes, yeast, and animal liver. In the laboratory, scientists can synthesize alpha-lipoic acid, which can then be given as an injection or formulated into tablets or capsules.

## USES

People with diabetes use alpha-lipoic acid to treat nerve damage to the hands and feet (called peripheral neuropathy). This painful nerve condition can cause various symptoms such as burning sensations in the feet and difficulty controlling movement. Oxidative stress is thought to play a role in the progression of diabetic nerve damage. As an anti-oxidant, alpha-lipoic acid may decrease oxidative stress and improve symptoms such as pain. However, there is no evidence that alpha-lipoic acid *prevents* diabetic nerve damage. In addition, studies have not shown that alpha-lipoic acid significantly decreases blood glucose levels.

Although alpha-lipoic acid has been used for several years in Germany, long-term trials in the United States are needed to determine whether alpha-lipoic acid slows progression or only improves symptoms of nerve damage. Much is still unknown about its use.

Alpha-lipoic acid is also used to treat many other conditions such as Parkinson's, Alzheimer's, cataracts, and glaucoma.

## DOSE

Typical doses of alpha-lipoic acid are 600 to 1,200 milligrams (mg) daily.

## STUDIES

Alpha-lipoic acid has been studied in a number of randomized, double-blind, placebo-controlled studies (the gold standard design of scientific studies). Overall, these studies have shown that alpha-lipoic acid decreases symptoms of painful diabetic nerve damage when compared to a placebo (dummy pill).

One series of studies is called the ALADIN (Alpha-Lipoic Acid in Diabetic Neuropathy) trials.

- In the first ALADIN study, 260 patients with type 2 diabetes and diabetic nerve damage were given an injection of alpha-lipoic acid in various doses (100, 600, or 1,200 mg) or a placebo once a day. The total symptoms of nerve damage decreased in those who were taking any dose of alpha-lipoic acid versus those who were taking a placebo. Burning, tingling, loss of sensation, and numbness decreased significantly in those patients on 600- or 1,200-mg versus a placebo. Pain scores decreased significantly only in the 600-mg group versus the placebo group. The neurodisability score, which measures vibration, pinprick, ankle reflexes, and temperature sensation in the big toe, decreased, but the decrease was significant only for the group taking 1,200-mg versus the placebo group. A1C, a measure of average blood glucose over 3 months, declined in all groups, but not significantly.

- In the second ALADIN study, 65 patients with type 1 or type 2 diabetes and nerve damage received an injection of alpha-lipoic acid or a placebo for 5 days. Then patients received a 600- or 1,200-mg tablet of alpha-lipoic acid or a placebo daily for 2 years. Researchers measured improvements in nerve damage in the patients. Patients taking either dose of alpha-lipoic acid had significant improvements versus the placebo group, although not for all types of nerve damage. The patients' neurodisability scores did not decrease, but the sample of patients may have been too small to detect changes. A1C did not decrease significantly, although A1C decreased from 9 percent to 8 percent after 2 years in the 1,200-mg group.

- The third ALADIN study examined 503 patients with type 2 diabetes. One group of patients received a 600-mg injection of alpha-lipoic acid for 3 weeks and then received either a 600-mg tablet of alpha-lipoic acid three times daily or a placebo for 6 months. The other group received a placebo "injection" for 3 weeks, followed by a placebo tablet for 6 months. Nerve damage impairment decreased after 19 days in both groups of patients who took alpha-lipoic acid versus the placebo. However, after 7 months, there was no significant difference in nerve damage scores between the groups.

- A separate study evaluated 120 patients who took alpha-lipoic acid 5 days a week for a total of 14 treatments. Symptoms declined significantly.

- A follow-up to this study evaluated three different doses of alpha-lipoic acid (600, 1,200, or 1,800 mg) versus a placebo for 5 weeks in 181 patients with diabetes. Total symptom scores declined significantly by 51 percent, 48 percent, and 52 percent, respectively, in the alpha-lipoic acid treatment groups versus 32 percent in the placebo group.

- Yet another study examined the results of a number of studies of alpha-lipoic acid in people with diabetic nerve disease. The study found that 53 percent of patients on alpha-lipoic acid versus 37 percent on a placebo had improved scores in their symptoms.

- The NATHAN I (Neurological Assessment of Thioctic Acid in Neuropathy) trial is an ongoing, long-term, multi-center trial in North America and Europe that is assessing the role of alpha-lipoic acid given orally for the prevention and treatment of diabetic neuropathy. A follow-up study called NATHAN II is currently investigating alpha-lipoic acid for relief of painful neuropathy symptoms, but as of this printing, the results have not yet been published.

## SIDE EFFECTS AND DRUG INTERACTIONS

To date, no serious side effects from alpha-lipoic acid have been reported, even though it has been used intravenously and in long-term trials. However, you may experience allergic reactions if you take alpha-lipoic acid. Alpha-lipoic acid may cause nausea and vomiting, as well as vertigo.

Anecdotal information indicates that alpha-lipoic acid may affect the thyroid, so ask your doctor whether you should have your thyroid levels tested. Studies in animals have shown that high doses of alpha-lipoic acid can be harmful when a thiamine deficiency is present. Ask your doctor about this side effect, particularly if you regularly drink large quantities of alcohol and may thus be thiamine-deficient. Your doctor may recommend that you take thiamine supplements; but ask your doctor first. Some anecdotal reports indicate that alpha-lipoic acid or other antioxidants may decrease the beneficial effects of chemotherapy, so also discuss this side effect with your doctor.

Monitor your blood glucose closely when taking alpha-lipoic acid and diabetes medications such as sulfonylureas. Low blood glucose can occur. In addition, you should not take alpha-lipoic acid and antacids at the same time because your body may not absorb the alpha-lipoic acid properly. Instead, space these medications a few hours apart.

# BANABA

## *Lagerstroemia speciosa*

Banaba is a type of crape myrtle that grows in the Philippines, India, Malaysia, and Australia. This tropical, flowering tree has bright pink to purple blooms that give way to nut-like fruits. Its leathery leaves turn red-orange in the fall. As part of folk medicine in the Philippines, banaba leaves are used to make a tea to treat diabetes.

## USES

Recently, banaba has become popular in the United States as a treatment for type 2 diabetes. Its leaves are used to make an oral form of the supplement, found as a single ingredient or as one of several ingredients in dietary supplements. Banaba's active ingredients are thought to stimulate cells to take up glucose and work similarly to insulin.

However, banaba's effect on blood glucose has not been confirmed in large, rigorous, long-term studies. Its effect on A1C, a measure of average blood glucose over 3 months, has never been reported. No information on its long-term use in people is available.

Banaba is used in multi-ingredient products for weight loss, though it has never been studied for this purpose in humans. Its potential for weight loss is based on studies in animals.

Banaba leaves are also used as a diuretic and purgative (used to empty the bowels) supplement. Its roots are used to treat upset stomach.

## Dose

In studies, scientists have used banaba in doses of 16–48 mg daily. The most effective dose in one small study was a daily 48-mg soft-gel capsule containing 1% corsolic acid.

## Studies

One very small study indicates that banaba may be helpful in lowering blood glucose in those with type 2 diabetes. However, the authors only reported percentage lowering of blood glucose and did not report the actual values.

- The study examined 10 patients with type 2 diabetes who took three different doses of banaba (16, 32, or 48 mg) in soft- or hard-gel capsules for 15 days. The patients stopped taking their regular diabetes medications 45 days before the study. At the end of the study, the patients taking the 32- and 48-mg soft gels showed an 11% and 30% decrease, respectively, in their basal blood glucose values. In addition, patients taking the 48-mg dose had a significant decrease of 20% in their basal blood glucose.

## Side Effects and Drug Interactions

No adverse effects or drug interactions with banaba have been reported. However, a person should be cautious about low blood glucose when taking banaba with diabetes medications or other dietary supplements that may lower blood glucose. As with any supplement, tell your doctor or pharmacist if you're planning to take or are taking banaba.

# BENFOTIAMINE

For many decades, neurological disorders such as diabetes and alcohol-related nerve damage have been treated with vitamin B1. However, vitamin B1, which is also called thiamine, is not absorbed by the body very well, and high levels are needed for successful treatment. Benfotiamine, a fat-soluble form of the vitamin, provides much higher levels of thiamine in the blood and tissues and thus may be more effective.

These vitamins are also called allithiamines because they are found in the *Allium* vegetable family, which includes garlic, onions, shallots, and leeks. Other foods that may contain thiamine include whole-grain cereals and breads, peas, beans, and nuts, as well as potatoes and certain meats (pork and liver). Consuming large quantities of raw freshwater fish and shellfish may decrease your level of thiamine.

## USES

Benfotiamine may relieve the effects of certain diabetes-related complications such as neuropathy (nerve damage), retinopathy (eye disease), and nephropathy (kidney disease). It may correct thiamine deficiencies in these conditions, even in people with end-stage renal (kidney) disease on dialysis.

Benfotiamine enhances the activity of an important enzyme

involved in glucose metabolism called transketolase. By enhancing this activity, it prevents glucose from being metabolized in a way that can cause damage. It may also diminish or even correct cell damage by normalizing cell division rates and decreasing apoptosis, or programmed cell death.

## Dose

The dose studied in diabetes-related neuropathy is 300–450 mg daily, administered in divided doses. For example, 100 or 150 mg benfotiamine three times a day. The dose used for alcohol-related neuropathy is higher.

## Studies

Most studies of benfotiamine have been done in people with diabetes and neuropathy.

- In a well-designed pilot study (randomized, double-blind, placebo-controlled), researchers studied 40 patients with neuropathy. Twenty patients received 100 mg of benfotiamine four times a day, and 20 patients received a placebo (dummy pill). After 3 weeks, neuropathy symptoms improved in the benfotiamine-treated group, although vibration-sensation scores did not improve.

- In another study, a preparation of 100 mg of benfotiamine plus other B vitamins was given four times a day to 30 neuropathy patients for 9 weeks, followed by a lower dose for 3 more weeks (50 mg four times a day). A control group of patients took a conventional B vitamin for the entire 12 weeks. The benfotiamine-treated patients had significant neuropathic pain relief and improvements in vibration perception (a sensation test), whereas the B-vitamin-only group had only minor improvements.

- Another 6-week study was conducted in 36 people with

diabetes and painful neuropathy. Twelve patients were given a combination of 80 mg of benfotiamine plus other B vitamins four times a day. Another group of 12 patients received a similar combination that contained only 40 mg of benfotiamine four times a day. The other 12 patients received a supplement containing only 50 mg of benfotiamine three times a day. All groups had improvements in pain relief and sensation, but the best results were reported in those patients taking the highest dose of benfotiamine.

- Another 12-week study, also with good study design, evaluated a supplement containing benfotiamine plus vitamins B6 and B12 in 24 patients. Thirteen patients received a placebo. Eleven patients received 80 mg of benfotiamine plus the B vitamins four times a day for 2 weeks, followed by 80 mg of benfotiamine three times a day for the remainder of the 12 weeks. Vibration perception and nerve conduction velocity (another test of sensation) improved in the benfotiamine group.

## SIDE EFFECTS AND DRUG INTERACTIONS

Benfotiamine appears to be a very safe dietary supplement. There are no reports of major side effects when used appropriately, though some people who are prone to allergies may have allergy-like skin rashes.

Certain herbs, such as betel nuts (Areca) and horsetail (Equisetum), may decrease the activity of thiamine and cause deficiencies. Antibiotics, oral contraceptives, and diuretics may decrease your body's natural thiamine levels. Also, the important diabetes drug metformin may decrease thiamine activity in the body. Other drugs, such as the seizure medicine phenytoin (Dilantin) and some chemotherapy drugs, may decrease the body's natural thiamine.

# BILBERRY
## *Vaccinium myrtillus*

This plant is a cousin of the American blueberry and huckleberry. Its little blue berries grow on shrubs in singles or pairs, unlike blueberries, which grow in clusters. Bilberries come from Northern and Central Europe, where they are still enjoyed today in jellies, pies, and cobblers. Historically, people have used bilberries to treat kidney stones and typhoid fever and induce menstruation. During World War II, British pilots were said to have eaten bilberry jam to improve their night vision. However, bilberry's benefit for night vision has not been demonstrated in recent studies.

## USES

People use two different forms of the bilberry plant in medicine: the dried berries and the leaves. Both forms are used to treat type 2 diabetes.

The berries are used to treat vision problems, such as retinopathy and cataracts, related to diabetes. Bilberries contain bioflavonoids, which are thought to strengthen blood vessels and improve blood flow. People soak the dried berries in water, then mash, strain, and drink the juices as a liquid. Alternately, bilberry leaves are used to make teas to treat diabetes. Some speculate that the chromium content of the leaves could help lower blood glucose, but this has never been studied.

Despite its popularity, there is very little evidence that bilberry is of any benefit to people with diabetes. Bilberry's effect on blood glucose has never been studied in humans. Preliminary evidence has shown that bilberry may help prevent cataracts, which may be important to people with diabetes because they are more prone to cataracts.

## DOSE

Standard daily doses are 20–60 grams (g) of dried, ripe berries. One study showed that taking 160 mg of bilberry extract twice a day improved retinopathy.

## STUDIES

There are no human studies in the United States related to bilberry use and diabetes.

- In one small study published in Italian, patients were given bilberry extract twice daily. The 23 patients had retinopathy related to diabetes or hypertension. The 11 patients on bilberry and 12 patients on a placebo were treated for 1 month. The bilberry group showed significant improvement in parameters that assess vision.

- A study of diabetic rats given bilberry leaves for 4 days resulted in consistent decreases in plasma glucose.

In spite of early enthusiasm and speculation during World War II about the beneficial effect of bilberry preserves in improving night vision in Royal Air Force pilots, this effect has not been shown in scientific studies.

- One randomized, double-blind, placebo-controlled study (the gold-standard design of scientific studies) was done in 15 men recruited from a naval air station. The subjects were given 160 mg of bilberry extract or a placebo three times a day for 21 days. The bilberry extract contained 25% antho-cyanosides, which are powerful antioxidants with specific benefits for eyes. There were no differences between the groups in night visual acuity or night contrast sensitivity.

- In another randomized, double-blind, placebo-controlled study, 16 men with normal vision were given three differ-ent doses of anthocyanosides (12, 24, or 36 mg) or a pla-cebo daily, with a 2-week washout between doses. There were no differences in night vision between the treatment and placebo groups.

- Another randomized, double-blind, placebo-controlled study evaluated three different night-vision tests in 18 healthy male volunteers. The subjects received 12 or 24 mg of anthocyanosides or a placebo twice daily for 4 days, with a 2-week washout between doses. Once again there was no difference between the treatment and placebo groups.

## SIDE EFFECTS AND DRUG INTERACTIONS

Bilberry is relatively benign, although high doses or prolonged use in animals have caused toxicity and death. Most reported adverse effects have been mild digestive distress, skin rashes, and drowsiness.

There are no known drug interactions. Yet, bilberry inhib-its the activity of platelets and thus interferes with clotting. Bilberry may interact with drugs or supplements that also pos-sess antiplatelet activity. Since bilberry may theoretically affect blood glucose, patients should monitor their blood glucose levels when taking bilberry along with diabetes medications. If an alcohol-based extract of bilberry is used, you may experi-ence a severe reaction, with symptoms that may include severe nausea, copious vomiting, flushing, head throbbing, vertigo, racing heart, blurred vision, and confusion.

# BITTER MELON
*Momordica charantia*

Bitter melon is a climbing plant with green, bumpy, cucumber-like fruits. The inside of the fruit is yellow with bright red coating around the seeds. Bitter melon is related to honeydew, Persian melon, cantaloupe, muskmelon, and casaba. It is cultivated as both food and medicine in various parts of the world, including India, Asia, Africa, and South America. It gets its name from its signature bitter taste.

Traditionally, bitter melon has been used to treat psoriasis, gastrointestinal disorders, kidney stones, and fever. As a topical agent, it's often used for wounds and infections. Women have used bitter melon to help induce menstruation and terminate pregnancies. Recently it has also been used to treat cancer and HIV.

## USES

People with type 1 or type 2 diabetes use the fruit and seeds of bitter melon. It can be consumed as a fruit, juice, or extract (the latter in tablet form). Bitter melon contains several chemical ingredients that are thought to lower blood glucose. However, most of the studies of bitter melon and diabetes have been small and poorly designed. Overall, bitter melon may be considered safe when eaten as a vegetable, but it is not consistently safe when used in supplement form.

## DOSE

There is no recommended dose, since people use various forms of the fruit, including juice, powder, vegetable pulp suspensions, and injections. One study indicated that the dose should be one small, unripe melon eaten daily or 50 to 100 milliliters (ml) fresh juice drunk daily with food. Bitter melon extract tablets are becoming increasingly available as well. One manufacturer stated the dose is 3 grams daily of 100% dried fruit.

## STUDIES

Few studies have evaluated bitter melon's effect on diabetes, and most have not had adequate study design to draw conclusive results.

- The largest study used an aqueous suspension of bitter melon vegetable pulp in 100 patients with type 2 diabetes. The authors did not state the amount of bitter melon used but stated that it was based on body weight. Bitter melon significantly reduced blood glucose levels in patients after a few hours. However, the long-term effects were not evaluated.

- In another study, bitter melon was prepared as an injectable "plant insulin" and injected in five patients with type 1 diabetes and six patients with type 2 diabetes. The dose was based on patients' blood glucose levels. A control group consisted of six patients with type 1 diabetes and two patients with type 2 diabetes who did not receive any bitter melon. Blood glucose was measured; then bitter melon was administered, and glucose was measured 4, 6, 8, and

12 hours after injection. In patients with type 1 diabetes, mean fasting glucose decreased 4 hours after injection and was maintained 6 and 8 hours after injection. In the patients with type 2 diabetes, there was no significant decline in blood glucose from baseline.

- A small study indicated that bitter melon may decrease A1C (a measure of average blood glucose over 3 months) after 7 weeks of use.

- A more recent study used appropriate study design to evaluate the effects of bitter melon on diabetes. Under strictly supervised conditions, 40 patients were randomly assigned to receive either bitter melon or a placebo (dummy pill). The researchers did not state the dose of bitter melon in the study but stated that two capsules were given three times a day for 3 months. The capsule was presumed to contain 100 percent dried fruit, although this was not confirmed by the researchers. In both the bitter melon and placebo groups, A1C increased slightly, although results were not significant. A few patients in the bitter melon group complained of abdominal discomfort, pain, and diarrhea.

## SIDE EFFECTS AND DRUG INTERACTIONS

The major side effect of bitter melon is stomach discomfort. However, some very serious, isolated events have occurred, including hypoglycemic coma from a tea containing bitter melon.

Young women of childbearing age should consumer bitter melon with caution, since it may induce menstruation and inadvertently cause miscarriage. Women who are breastfeeding should not use bitter melon because there have been no studies for this group.

Children should not use bitter melon, since serious adverse effects have occurred, including hypoglycemic coma. Individuals of Mediterranean or Middle-Eastern descent with known G6PDH deficiency or those who have allergies to the melon family should also avoid bitter melon.

Bitter melon may cause low blood glucose when combined with traditional diabetes medications such as sulfonylureas. Tell your doctor if you are taking or are considering taking bitter melon.

# BLONDE PSYLLIUM

*Plantago ovata*

Psyllium is a soluble fiber found in everything from Metamucil to whole-grain cereals. It grows in various parts of the world, including India, the Middle East, Spain, and the United States. The tiny seeds and seed husks of this grain are used as an ingredient in laxatives and foods. Although psyllium is probably best known for treating constipation, it has recently garnered attention as an ingredient in cereals that may help lower cholesterol and reduce the risk of heart disease. Blonde psyllium is the most common variety, although there is also black psyllium.

## USES

People with type 2 diabetes use psyllium to reduce their post-prandial (post-meal) blood glucose. Although readily available as a nonprescription medication, psyllium has not been approved for treating diabetes and is therefore considered a potential supplement for lowering blood glucose.

Some researchers theorize that when psyllium comes in contact with water during digestion, it forms a gel that slows the small intestine's absorption of glucose. This could decrease blood glucose levels after meals. Other researchers suggest that psyllium may delay gastric emptying (the rate at which food empties from your stomach) or slow carbohydrates' access to digestive enzymes. Some studies have demonstrated that taking psyllium leads to lower post-meal glucose levels, even if the meal is eaten several hours after the fiber was taken. This is known as the "second-meal effect." In psyllium, the soluble fiber may trigger a lower post-meal increase in insulin that leads to a smaller glucose counter-response.

The FDA allows foods that contain at least 1.7 g psyllium to claim that they can reduce heart disease as part of a low-fat and low-cholesterol diet. However, the American Heart Association has not included psyllium as part of a stepwise dietary approach. Psyllium may lower cholesterol by absorbing dietary fats.

## Dose

In studies, scientists have used 5.1 g psyllium twice or three times daily to lower postmeal glucose. Scientists have also used 5.1 g psyllium twice daily or 3.4 g psyllium three times daily to lower cholesterol.

## Studies

Several small studies have demonstrated the benefit of psyllium in reducing post-meal glucose and cholesterol.

- In one study, 18 patients with type 2 diabetes received either psyllium or a placebo (dummy pill) twice daily before a standardized breakfast and supper. Patients' blood glucose was measured at baseline for each of two 15-hour phases, and post-meal values were measured every 15 minutes for 2 hours, then once after 30 minutes and hourly thereafter for 2.5 hours more. A 7-day wash-out was followed by a second test period when patients were crossed over to the opposite group. The scientists reported that peak post-meal glucose levels were 14 percent lower with psyllium versus a placebo after breakfast, and 21 percent lower with psyllium versus a placebo after dinner. However, these results should be viewed with caution because the numbers did not achieve statistical significance, and the authors did not state specific glucose values. The scientists reported that post-lunch glucose levels were reduced even further by 31 percent. It was speculated that this was a "second-meal," or residual, effect of the psyllium.

- One of the largest studies of psyllium was a double-blind, placebo-controlled trial in 125 patients with type 2 diabetes who participated in dietary therapy for 6 weeks and then took 5 g psyllium or a placebo three times daily for 6 weeks. Mean plasma glucose values declined 6 weeks after diet treatment. After an additional 6 weeks of psyllium, mean plasma glucose declined even further. The scientists stated that there was a significant difference between the psyllium group and the placebo group. Mean LDL cholesterol also declined after 6 weeks of psyllium use.

- Another well-designed study assessed 34 men with type 2 diabetes for 10 weeks. Following a 2-week dietary stabilization phase, the patients were randomized to 5.1 g psyllium or a placebo twice daily. All-day mean plasma glucose was 11% lower in the psyllium-treated group. Post-lunch glucose was 19% lower in the psyllium-treated group. LDL cholesterol decreased by 4.7% in the psyllium group and increased by 8.3% in the placebo group, but this difference was not statistically significant. Total cholesterol decreased by 2.1% in the psyllium group and increased by 6.9% in the placebo group—a statistically significant difference.

# SIDE EFFECTS AND DRUG INTERACTIONS

Allergic reactions, including cough and sinusitis, have been reported, as well as adverse gastrointestinal effects, including flatulence. The inner seed parts may be responsible for the allergic reactions. People may develop swallowing disorders due to obstruction of the esophagus with psyllium. Individuals with phenylketonuria may have problems if a psyllium supplement is sweetened with aspartame. People with diabetes should also be cautious that psyllium products contain sugar, which could increase blood glucose.

There are a variety of drug interactions, mainly due to medications binding with psyllium molecules and decreasing the absorption of these medications when taken at the same time as the supplement. This includes decreased absorption of carbamazepine, iron supplements, and riboflavin.

On the other hand, taking psyllium with diabetes and cholesterol-lowering medications may increase the effectiveness of these drugs. For example, some individuals taking psyllium along with statins and other cholesterol-lowering drugs have improved their cholesterol levels. Taking psyllium may relieve the stomach discomfort of drugs such as orlistat and misoprostol. As with any supplement, tell your doctor if you are taking or are planning to take psyllium.

# CAIAPO

## *Ipomoea batatas*

Caiapo comes from a white sweet potato cultivated in a mountainous region in the Kagawa Prefecture of Japan. It is eaten raw to treat diabetes, hypertension, and anemia. The potato also grows in the mountains of South America, and it reportedly has been used by Native Americans to treat thirst, weight loss, and symptoms of diabetes.

## USES

Caiapo is not very well known in the United States. However, an extract of the caiapo potato skin is used to treat type 2 diabetes in Japan. It is unclear exactly how caiapo may lower blood glucose, but scientists speculate that it improves insulin sensitivity and decreases insulin resistance. Its long-term effects have never been studied in people.

## DOSE

Preliminary information from a small study found that 4 grams (g) daily before breakfast may help treat type 2 diabetes.

## STUDIES

There have been two small studies of caiapo in patients with type 2 diabetes.

- A 6-week pilot study of 18 patients with type 2 diabetes compared a low dose of caiapo (2 g), a high dose of caiapo (4 g), and a placebo (dummy pill). Fasting blood glucose decreased from 158 to 151 milligrams/deciliter (mg/dl) with low-dose caiapo and from 149 to 130 mg/dl with high-dose caiapo. The low dose did not reduce patients' A1C, a measure of average blood glucose over 3 months. A1C values decreased slightly in the high-dose group, but it was not a significant difference. Total and LDL cholesterol also decreased in patients on the higher dose.

- A well-designed study (randomized, double-blind, placebo-controlled) examined 61 patients with type 2 diabetes for 3 months. Most patients were treating their diabetes through diet alone. Thirty patients received 4 g of caiapo daily and 31 patients received a placebo. A1C declined from 7.2% to 6.7% in those taking caiapo but increased from 7.0% to 7.1% in the placebo group. In the caiapo group, fasting blood glucose declined from 144 to 129 mg/dl and 2-hour post-meal glucose declined from 193 to 163 mg/dl. Cholesterol was significantly lower in the caiapo group than in the placebo group. Weight also decreased by 3.7 kilograms (roughly 8 pounds) in the caiapo group after 3 months. Blood pressure levels did not change.

## SIDE EFFECTS AND DRUG INTERACTIONS

Most side effects are gastrointestinal in nature and include constipation, stomach pain, flatulence, and gas. In theory, caiapo may cause low blood glucose if used with diabetes medications or other dietary supplements that lower blood glucose. Tell your doctor if you are taking or are considering taking caiapo. Check your blood glucose frequently to make sure that it is not too low. And monitor your A1C levels at 3-month intervals.

# CHIA
## *Salvia Hispanica*

Chia has recently become popular as a dietary supplement for diabetes. The word chia comes from an Aztec word meaning oily. The Latin American plant is part of the mint family and grows to about one meter in height with purple or white flowers that form clusters on the stem. It is famous as the "chia pets" that are sprouts grown on clay figures. Chia seeds have recently become popular and have been described on television and the Internet as a "super food."

## USES

Chia seeds are used in supplements and also added to foods. The seeds contain a plant source of omega-3 fatty acids, which is alpha-linolenic acid. They also contain fiber, protein, calcium, magnesium, iron, and antioxidants. The seeds have been described as having a nutty, agreeable flavor. Some patients with diabetes eat chia seeds to decrease their post-meal glucose, an effect that may occur because of the seeds' high content of soluble fiber.

## DOSE

A recent study has used 37 grams (g) daily of chia. However, chia seeds may be sprinkled liberally on salads, soup, or yogurt.

Some Internet sources recommend using a few teaspoonfuls on food every day.

## STUDIES

A single study has described the use of chia in people with diabetes. Controversy has stemmed over whether black or white chia seeds are better. Some individuals recommend black chia seeds because they are less expensive than white chia seeds. The study described below used white chia seeds in the form of a specific manufactured product called Salba.

- In the study, 20 patients with type 2 diabetes were randomly selected to receive a daily dose of 37 g a day of chia or a wheat bran placebo (dummy pill). The researchers knew that the patients were taking chia, but the patients did not know. After 12 weeks, the patients were crossed over to the other group after a washout period of 4–6 weeks. In the chia group, patients' A1C levels (a measure of average blood glucose over 3 months) declined significantly from 6.9 to 6.7% but did not change in the placebo group (6.9% at the beginning and after 12 weeks). Systolic blood pressure declined significantly in the chia group from 129 to 123 mmHg but increased from 122 to 129 mmHg in the placebo group. Diastolic blood pressure also decreased in the chia group, but the change was not significant (81 to 78 mmHg). Diastolic blood pressure increased in the placebo group (76 to 79 mmHg). Other indicators of cardiovascular disease also improved in the chia group.

## SIDE EFFECTS AND DRUG INTERACTIONS

Side effects of chia include increases in triglycerides in people who already have high triglycerides. However, the study using

Salba did not show increased triglycerides in participants. Another potential caution is that high dietary intake of alpha-linolenic acid may increase the risk for advanced prostate cancer, so men with pre-existing prostate cancer should avoid chia seeds. Lab tests of total cholesterol, kidney function, or the ability to clot blood have not shown any adverse effects from chia.

# CHROMIUM

Chromium is a chemical element that comes in several different forms. In nutrition, the important form is a mineral found in foods such as high-bran cereals, whole grains, broccoli, egg yolks, brewer's yeast, meat, nuts, cheese, beer, and wine. It is unclear exactly how much chromium the average person should consume, but scientists at the Institute of Medicine have set a minimum daily requirement of 35 micrograms (mcg) a day for young men and 25 mcg a day for young women.

Chromium deficiencies can occur in pregnant women, people with poor diets, or people with poor glucose control or high glucose intake. There is currently no evidence that chromium deficiency rates are higher in people with diabetes than in those without diabetes. However, in studies, animals with chromium deficiencies have developed diabetes. It is difficult to determine when someone has a chromium deficiency as there is no good test available for measuring levels of chromium in the body. Unfortunately, this also makes it challenging to measure how chromium supplements affect chromium deficiencies.

## USES

People with type 1 or type 2 diabetes use chromium to improve their blood glucose and cholesterol levels. A form called chromium picolinate, which comes in tablets or capsules, appears to be the most appropriate product. Chromium is also used for weight loss and to reverse steroid-induced diabetes.

Scientists know that the human body needs chromium to metabolize glucose. However, no one knows exactly how it affects blood glucose. It may enhance the effects of insulin or the activity of insulin-producing cells in the pancreas.

In August 2005, the U.S. Food and Drug Administration authorized a qualified health claim that chromium picolinate may reduce the risk of insulin resistance, based on a small study. The official American Diabetes Association stance is that there is no conclusive evidence to support the use of chromium supplements in diabetes. However, its popularity continues, and overall side effects have not been serious.

## DOSE

The Food and Nutrition Board of the Institute of Medicine has determined an adequate intake of 35 mcg daily for young men and 25 mcg daily for young women. No upper limit for chromium intake has been established because few serious adverse effects have been reported. A typical dose of chromium is 200 mcg daily, although higher doses have been studied and shown to be more effective.

## STUDIES

Studies of chromium for treating blood glucose have had mixed results. Part of the problem has been controversy about the most appropriate formulation for chromium or the best markers for measuring chromium in the body.

- In a well-designed study (randomized, double-blind, placebo-controlled) of 180 Chinese patients, fasting blood glucose decreased significantly in patients taking 1,000 mcg daily of chromium picolinate. A1C levels, a measure of average blood glucose over 3 months, also decreased. This was compared to patients taking 200 mcg daily chromium picolinate or a placebo (dummy pill). In the study, patients received 100 mcg chromium picolinate, 500 mcg chromium picolinate, or a placebo twice daily for 4 months. Fasting glucose decreased significantly in the 1,000-mcg group at 2 and 4 months. From graph interpretation, A1C was 9.4% in the two chromium groups and 9.2% in the placebo group at the beginning of the study. After 4 months, A1C was 8.5%, 7.5%, and 6.6%, respectively, in the placebo, 200 mcg, and 1,000 mcg groups. Thus, A1C decreased by 2.8% in the highest dose group and by 1.9% in the other chromium group. However, people should keep in mind that the Chinese patients in this study may have had different dietary chromium intake than average Americans. The Chinese patients were also much leaner than many typical diabetes patients in the United States.

- A recent analysis of several chromium and diabetes studies found that the data are inconclusive and more studies are needed to evaluate the role of chromium supplementation in diabetes.

- Another review evaluated several studies, including those with long-term use of chromium in higher doses, and found that, overall, there may be some benefit to using chromium supplements.

- Two recent studies have shown negative results. One study used 800 mcg chromium picolinate daily for 3 months in patients with impaired glucose tolerance, and the other study used 1,000 mcg chromium picolinate daily in obese, type 2 diabetes patients who took insulin. However, critics have stated that the chromium dose used was less than optimal because the chromium picolinate used contained only 12.4% chromium picolinate.

- Supplements containing chromium picolinate in combination with the B vitamin biotin are undergoing extensive study. For example, a well-designed study (randomized, double-blind, placebo-controlled) of people with type 2 diabetes who take oral diabetes medications showed positive results on blood glucose. A total of 226 patients took a supplement containing 600 mcg chromium plus 2 mg of biotin, and 122 patients took a placebo daily for 90 days. In the chromium group, A1C decreased by 0.54% from a baseline of 8.73%, whereas the placebo group decreased by 0.34% from a baseline of 8.46%. Overall fasting glucose also decreased significantly from 170 to 160 milligrams/deciliter (mg/dl) in the chromium group and increased slightly in the placebo group from 171 to 172 mg/dl.

## SIDE EFFECTS AND DRUG INTERACTIONS

Side effects related to higher-than-recommended doses of chromium include kidney toxicity, severe illness (due to breakdown of red blood cells), decreased number of platelets, and liver malfunction. Other adverse effects have included skin reactions and mood disturbances. However, studies have demonstrated the safety of large doses and long-term usage of chromium picolinate.

There are unique effects of other drugs on chromium. Steroids may deplete chromium. Histamine blockers, such as the over-the-counter medication Pepcid, and proton pump inhibitors, such as the over-the-counter medication Prilosec, may block chromium absorption. Certain drugs and vitamins, such as anti-inflammatory drugs (ibuprofen) and vitamin C, may increase chromium absorption. Taking chromium together with zinc may decrease the absorption of both nutrients. Finally, low blood glucose is a possibility when taking chromium with insulin or other diabetes drugs.

# CINNAMON

## *Cinnamomum cassia* or *Cinnamomum aromaticum*

**M**ost people are familiar with cinnamon as a popular flavor in foods, beverages, and things like chewing gum and mouthwash. However, cinnamon is also a trendy supplement for treating blood glucose in type 1 and type 2 diabetes.

Chinese cinnamon, which is called cassia, is the variety used for diabetes. Cinnamon comes from an evergreen tree that grows over 20 feet high and has a white, aromatic bark and angular branches. It has leaves about 7 inches long and small, yellow flowers that bloom in early summer. The tree grows in tropical climates, and the bark is removed in short lengths and dried. Both cinnamon bark and flowers are used in medicine.

### USES

Cinnamon is used for type 1 and type 2 diabetes and for gastrointestinal complaints such as indigestion or gas. Scientists think that the active ingredients in cinnamon may increase insulin sensitivity.

### DOSE

Scientists have used does of 1, 3, or 6 grams (g) daily of *Cinnamomum cassia* in divided doses. One gram of cinnamon is roughly equivalent to a half teaspoonful, which may be used in cereals, beverages, breads, and other foods.

# STUDIES

Studies have not consistently shown that cinnamon reduces A1C, a measure of average blood glucose over 3 months. High doses of cinnamon have been effective in treating blood glucose in studies in Pakistan, but the same benefits have not been shown in studies in Germany or in the United States.

- A study in Pakistan found that cinnamon improved glucose and blood fats, called lipids, in 60 people with type 2 diabetes who were taking sulfonylurea medications, such as glipizide or glyburide. Patients were given 1, 3, or 6 g per day cinnamon or a placebo (dummy pill) for 40 days. Fasting blood glucose declined by 18–29% after 40 days in all three groups. At a dose of 1 g, glucose decreased from a baseline of 209 to 157 milligrams/deciliter (mg/dl); at 3 g, glucose decreased from 205 to 169 mg/dl; and at 6 g, glucose decreased from 234 to 166 mg/dl. Cinnamon was withheld for the next 20 days, and fasting glucose was still lower than at the beginning of the study, indicating that cinnamon had a sustained benefit. Improvements in lipids were also significant. Total cholesterol decreased by 12–26%, triglycerides decreased by 23–30%, and LDL cholesterol also declined by 7–27%. HDL cholesterol did not improve, and the authors did not report changes in A1C.

- Another study was done in Germany in 79 individuals with type 2 diabetes. The study was well designed (randomized, double-blind, placebo-controlled) and lasted 4 months. Scientists used an aqueous cinnamon extract that was thought to be less allergenic than other forms. Patients were randomized to receive either a placebo or a capsule containing 1 g cinnamon three times a day. In the cinnamon group, mean baseline fasting glucose decreased by 10%, from 167 to 147 mg/dl. In the placebo group, mean baseline fasting glucose decreased by 3%, from 156 to 150 mg/dl. A1C did not decrease significantly in either the cinnamon or placebo groups. There were no differences in lipids levels.

- Another study examined the effects of cinnamon in 25 post-menopausal women with type 2 diabetes taking oral diabetes medications. The patients were given 1.5 g cinnamon daily or a placebo for 6 weeks. There were no significant differences between either group in A1C or fasting blood glucose.

- A separate study of 72 adolescents with type 1 diabetes found no improvements in A1C with cinnamon. The patients were given 1 g cinnamon or a placebo for 90 days. There were no changes in insulin doses for patients.

- A well-designed, 3-month study in the United States of 57 patients with type 2 diabetes showed no significant changes in A1C, fasting lipids, or insulin levels between 1 g of cinnamon daily or a placebo.

- An analysis of the five studies mentioned above of cinnamon in a total of 282 patients found that A1C did not decline significantly, although potential benefits in individual studies included decreases in fasting glucose and lipids, though not in significant amounts.

## SIDE EFFECTS AND DRUG INTERACTIONS

Side effects are rare and include possible skin rashes or irritation. Because cinnamon contains an ingredient that thins the blood, bleeding may occur if it is taken with blood-thinning medications or supplements. In theory, cinnamon may lower blood glucose if combined with diabetes medications such as sulfonylureas or insulin.

# COENZYME Q10

Coenzyme Q10 is a vitamin-like substance found in all cells. It is made by the body and is highly concentrated in the brain, heart, liver, kidneys, and pancreas. Coenzyme Q10 levels decrease with age and with certain disorders such as heart disease, Parkinson's disease, cancer, and periodontal disease. Coenzyme Q10 is found in foods such as poultry, beef, and broccoli. Scientists can formulate coenzyme Q10 into pills in the laboratory through special processes combining beets, sugarcane, and yeast.

## USES

There is some evidence that coenzyme Q10 may lower blood glucose *slightly*. Coenzyme Q10 is essential for cells to produce energy. Scientists theorize that, in diabetes, insulin-producing cells in the pancreas may not have the best possible coenzyme Q10 activity. In theory, taking coenzyme Q10 supplements may improve your body's ability to produce insulin.

Coenzyme Q10 is better known for its potential cardiovascular benefits. Most people take coenzyme Q10 to help treat a variety of diseases such as heart disease, Parkinson's, muscular dystrophy, and periodontal disease. Patients who take a class of cholesterol-lowering drugs called statins may take coenzyme

Q10 supplements because statins are thought to lower coenzyme Q10 levels. However, the benefit of taking coenzyme Q10 for this purpose has not been consistently shown in rigorous, long-term studies.

## DOSE

Doses of coenzyme Q10 have varied in different studies. In diabetes studies, the dose is 100–200 milligrams (mg) daily. For high blood pressure and other cardiovascular diseases, the dose has ranged from 100 to 225 mg daily, although up to 600 mg in divided doses has been used for various cardiovascular diseases.

## STUDIES

Even though there is much enthusiasm for coenzyme Q10, and long-term studies have not shown harmful effects, further long-term studies are needed to determine its place in daily therapy.

Coenzyme Q10 has been evaluated most extensively as a treatment for heart disease, including high blood pressure and congestive heart failure. People with diabetes need to be extra careful about their risk of heart disease as two out of three people with diabetes die from heart disease and stroke.

However, many of the studies have used an open-label study design, where the participants know what treatment they are receiving, which may result in an unintentional bias in favor of coenzyme Q10. Other studies have not used a control group. In still other trials, study design has been inadequate (lacking randomization or blinding), or the end results for patients have been unsatisfactory. For example, blood pressure studies have had unacceptable end points (the target result or desired effect sought in a study). Although systolic and diastolic blood pressures decreased significantly, the pressures achieved at the end of the study were still much higher than would be recommended for people with diabetes.

- In a study of 109 patients with high blood pressure, coenzyme Q10 was added to existing treatment with high blood pressure medications. The average dose was 225 mg per day, and patients were followed for an average of 13 months. Systolic pressure decreased from 159 to 147 mmHg, and diastolic pressure decreased from 94 to 85 mmHg.

- In a separate study, 30 patients with high blood pressure received 60 mg coenzyme Q10 twice a day, and 30 patients received a vitamin B complex for 8 weeks. In patients treated with coenzyme Q10, blood pressure decreased significantly from 168 to 152 mmHg systolic and 106 to 97 mmHg diastolic. Meanwhile, in patients treated with vitamin B, systolic blood pressure decreased from only 166 to 164 mmHg and diastolic blood pressure decreased from only 105 to 103 mmHg. Although the scientists reported that patients did not have diabetes, patients were thought to have insulin resistance. Baseline glucose decreased in the coenzyme Q10 group from 141 to 95 milligram/deciliter (mg/dl) after 8 weeks. Decreases in blood glucose in the vitamin B complex–treated group were not significant. Fasting plasma insulin decreased from 465 to 257 picomoles/liter in the coenzyme Q10 group. This did not change significantly in the vitamin B group.

- For congestive heart failure, the benefits of coenzyme Q10 are controversial. In general, coenzyme Q10 has improved the number of hospitalizations and certain clinical parameters of heart failure. In a well-designed, year-long study of 641 patients with heart failure, patients had fewer hospitalizations for heart failure and fewer episodes of pulmonary edema (excess fluid in the lungs) with coenzyme Q10. However, a recent study with excellent study design and well-defined parameters found no benefit with coenzyme Q10 in 55 patients with symptoms of serious heart failure. An ongoing long-term outcome trial with over 500 people with symptoms of heart failure who will be followed for over 2 years will hopefully better define the role of coenzyme Q10.

In studies of patients with type 1 or type 2 diabetes, coenzyme Q10 supplements have shown neutral to slightly improved effects on fasting glucose and A1C (a measure of blood glucose levels over 3 months).

- In a well-designed study, 34 patients with type 1 diabetes received 100 mg per day of coenzyme Q10 or a placebo (dummy pill) for 3 months. A1C decreased from 8.04 to 7.86% in the coenzyme Q10 group and from 8.02 to 7.84% in the placebo group. The decreases were not statistically significant in either group. Daily blood glucose decreased from 160 to 145 mg/dl in the coenzyme Q10 group and from 161 to 153 mg/dl in the placebo group. Again, the decreases were not significant in either group. There were no significant differences in systolic or diastolic blood pressures in either group.

- In a separate, well-designed study, 12 patients with type 2 diabetes were given 100 mg of coenzyme Q10 twice a day. Eleven patients received a placebo pill. All participants were also taking sulfonylureas, such as glyburide or glipizide. There was no improvement in diabetes control. A1C increased from 8.7 to 9.1% after 6 months in the coenzyme Q10 group and from 7.9 to 8.1% in the placebo group. Fasting glucose decreased from 211 to 198 mg/dl in the coenzyme Q10 group and from 203 to 191 mg/dl in the placebo group.

- Another study assessed the effect of coenzyme Q10 on blood glucose and blood pressure in 74 patients with type 2 diabetes and high cholesterol. Patients received either 100 mg of coenzyme Q10 twice daily, 200 mg fenofibrate daily, a combination of coenzyme Q10 and fenofibrate, or a placebo for 12 weeks. Blood glucose results were better for the combination of coenzyme Q10 and fenofibrate than either coenzyme Q10 alone or a placebo. The combination group may have benefited from the effect of fenofibrate on triglyceride lowering. The authors also reported that systolic pressure declined by 6.1 mmHg and diastolic pressure decreased by 2.9 mmHg with coenzyme Q10 supplementation.

## SIDE EFFECTS AND DRUG INTERACTIONS

Adverse effects have been rare, even with long-term use of up to 6 years. In a few patients, gastrointestinal problems, including diarrhea, nausea, anorexia, and epigastric distress, have occurred. Although early reports stated there were abnormal increases in certain liver function tests, long-term administration of 600 mg per day has not changed liver function.

Coenzyme Q10 may interfere with the efficacy of certain medications such as the blood-thinning drug warfarin. However, a study of patients taking coenzyme Q10 and warfarin did not show that taking the two together interferes with blood thinning. Smoking also depletes the body's coenzyme Q10 levels.

Treatment with statins may decrease levels of coenzyme Q10 that may contribute to statin-related muscle pain or aches, though this interaction is controversial. A study that used low doses of certain statins did not result in lower coenzyme Q10 levels, but another study using a low and high dose statin did find lower levels of coenzyme Q10. Decreased coenzyme Q10 concentrations with statin treatment have also been reported in people with diabetes.

People who take red-yeast rice should be aware that the supplement contains an ingredient that is essentially a statin and thus has statin-like effects. Red yeast may decrease the body's natural supply of coenzyme Q10.

On the other hand, taking coenzyme Q10 with blood pressure or diabetes medications may increase the effectiveness of these drugs. A potentially beneficial drug interaction has occurred with a cancer medication called doxorubicin. Taking coenzyme Q10 may decrease some of doxorubicin's harmful effects on the heart.

Some scientists say that coenzyme Q10 may have added benefit when combined with another supplement called L-carnitine to help provide anti-oxidant protection against certain toxins.

# FENUGREEK
## *Trigonella foenum-graecum*

Fenugreek is a green leafy herb that grows well in India, Egypt, and other parts of the Middle East. The plant was first described in Egypt in 1500 BC. Throughout history, it has been used to treat digestive problems, relieve symptoms of menopause, and induce lactation after childbirth.

Fenugreek leaves are eaten as a vegetable in India. Yet, in most parts of the world, the fragrant fenugreek seeds are used as a spice or medicine. The seeds smell and taste a bit like maple syrup, and they have been used to mask the taste of medicines.

### USES

The U.S. Food and Drug Administration has given fenugreek GRAS (Generally Recognized As Safe) status. Fenugreek seed is ground and taken by mouth to treat both type 1 and type 2 diabetes. However, there are few studies confirming how well it actually works. Fenugreek may help tissues in the pancreas and may improve glucose and carbohydrate absorption, as well as insulin resistance.

Fenugreek is also used to treat constipation and high cholesterol, and to promote lactation. However, there are no studies supporting its use in lactation.

## Dose

Doses vary, but a typical amount is 10–15 grams (g) daily, as a single dose or divided with meals, or 1 g of a hydroalcoholic extract.

## Studies

There have been only a few published studies on fenugreek and diabetes. Most of these were short-term, involved very few patients, and did not adequately report details.

- In one study, 10 patients with type 1 diabetes on insulin were included in a 10-day evaluation. The patients were assigned to either a placebo (dummy pill) or twice-daily 50 g fenugreek defatted seed powder used in unleavened bread. Fasting glucose decreased from an average of 272 to 196 milligrams/deciliter (mg/dl) in the fenugreek group. Total cholesterol, LDL, and triglycerides all decreased in the fenugreek group.

- A larger study involved a 6-month trial of fenugreek in 60 patients with poorly controlled type 2 diabetes. Fenugreek seed powder was given in two equal doses at lunch and dinner for a total of 25 g daily. Average fasting glucose decreased from 151 to 112 mg/dl after 6 months. Glucose values after meals also declined. Mean baseline 1-hour glucose was 245 mg/dl at the start of the study and decreased to 196 mg/dl after 6 months. Mean 2-hour glucose decreased from 257 to 171 mg/dl. Average A1C, a measure of average blood glucose over 3 months, decreased from 9.6 to 8.4% after 8 weeks.

- In a different study, 25 newly diagnosed type 2 diabetes patients were given a hydroalcoholic fenugreek extract or a placebo and instructed to continue their normal diet and exercise for 2 months. The group assigned to fenugreek was given 1 g daily of the seed extract. The fenugreek group did not differ from the placebo group in fasting or post-meal glucose, although this group had an improved lipid profile for triglycerides and HDL.

## SIDE EFFECTS AND DRUG INTERACTIONS

The main side effects include diarrhea and gas, or flatulence, which usually subsides after a few days. Pregnant women should not take fenugreek, since they may experience uterine contractions. People have reported runny nose, wheezing, and fainting after inhaling the seed powder. A patient with chronic asthma who applied fenugreek paste to the skin experienced wheezing and facial swelling. In theory, people with a peanut allergy may be allergic to fenugreek because it is part of the Leguminosae family. All of these side effects may occur in the infants of nursing mothers who use fenugreek, since fenugreek may be secreted in milk.

Patients who take anti-inflammatory drugs, blood-thinning drugs such as warfarin, or herbs that have blood-thinning effects, such as ginkgo biloba, garlic, or ginger should not use fenugreek. Fenugreek may also enhance the activity of diabetes medications and cause low blood glucose. As with any supplement, tell your doctor if you are taking or planning to take fenugreek.

# FISH OIL

Fish can be a healthy addition to your diet—and fish oil is one of the reasons why. Fish oil is an essential fatty acid, which means that we need to get it from our food instead of making it in our bodies. Essential fatty acids come in two main forms: omega-3 and omega-6. Fish oil is an omega-3 fatty acid, while gamma-linolenic acid is an omega-6 fatty acid (discussed later in this book).

Omega-3 fatty acids get their name because of their chemical structure. They have a double bond at their third carbon atom. There are two sources of omega-3 fatty acids: plant oils and fish oils. Fish oil contains the fatty acids eicosapentanoic acid (EPA) and docosahexanoic acid (DHA). It also contains long-chain polyunsaturated fatty acids. Good sources are salmon, trout, halibut, mackerel, sturgeon, tuna, and sardines. Omega-3 plant oils contains alpha linolenic acid, a substance that may help reduce cholesterol and reduce inflammation. The best sources of omega-3 plant oil are walnuts, flaxseed (linseed), canola, soybeans, and olives.

## USES

Omega-3 fish oil (containing the combination of EPA and DHA) has shown more cardiovascular health benefits than omega-3 plant oil (containing alpha linolenic acid). Fish oil is best known for treating cardiovascular disease, specifically high cholesterol. Scientists think that it may inhibit inflammation and the formation of clots in blood vessels. They first noticed the benefits of fish oil because people who ate a lot of fish tended to have low rates of cardiovascular disease. Since cardiovascular disease is the primary cause of death in diabetes, people with diabetes have become interested in using fish oil to reduce their risk of heart disease and stroke.

There is some interest in fish oil for prevention of type 2 diabetes. However, at this time, there is no evidence that fish oil can be used for this purpose. People with type 2 diabetes who have elevated cholesterol may benefit from taking fish oil.

Other uses include high blood pressure treatment (in higher-than-recommended doses) and ischemic stroke prevention. Fish oil is used to treat various inflammatory diseases, such as rheumatoid arthritis, psoriasis, inflammatory bowel disease, and skin inflammation. Individuals have also used fish oil for asthma, renal disease, and psychiatric disorders.

## Dose

The American Diabetes Association and the American Heart Association have recommended eating two servings per week of fish that are high in omega-3 fatty acids. Other sources of omega-3 fatty acids include fortified eggs and microalgae-derived oils.

For treating very high triglycerides, the American Heart Association recommends doses of 2 to 4 grams (g) a day. High triglyceride levels, which commonly occur in people with diabetes, can damage the pancreas. A prescription product called Lovaza contains 375 milligrams (mg) DHA and 465 mg EPA. It is approved for treating high cholesterol, so ask your doctor if you're interested in this product.

When buying a nonprescription fish oil supplement, it is important to look for the *total* amount of EPA and DHA. Most supplements contain only 200–400 mg of EPA plus DHA per capsule. Therefore, you may have to take as many as 12–16 capsules of fish oil to obtain the equivalent of one capsule of the prescription product Lovaza. However, more concentrated dietary supplements containing higher doses of EPA and DHA are being formulated. The American Heart Association recommends 1g per day of EPA plus DHA for people who have cardiovascular disease. There is emerging evidence that people at risk of cardiovascular disease should also take fish oil. Although the exact amount is not known, a common recommendation is 250–500 mg daily of EPA plus DHA.

## STUDIES

Numerous studies have assessed fish oil for treatment of cardiovascular disease and other disorders, including diabetes.

- One of the largest studies evaluated fish oil supplementation as a means to prevent second heart attacks in 11,324 individuals who had already suffered a heart attack. In the study (called GISSI), patients were randomized to daily doses of 1 g per day of omega-3 fatty acid, 300 mg of vitamin E, a combination of omega-3 fatty acid and vitamin E, or a placebo (dummy pill). After 3 1/2 years, the omega-3 fatty acid group had a 10% reduction in deaths, heart attacks, and strokes. Cardiovascular death was lowered by 17% and overall mortality went down by 14%. There was no benefit seen in the vitamin E group. Although 15% of the subjects had diabetes, the researchers did not report the results specifically for this group.

- A separate study assessed how long it would take to achieve benefit in the GISSI trial and found that the risk of total mortality was significantly reduced after 3 months of treatment and that the risk of sudden death was significantly reduced after 4 months of treatment.

- The Cochrane Collaboration published a review of randomized trials in people with type 2 diabetes that compared fish oil to a placebo or vegetable oil. The study looked at the effects of taking fish oil supplements on fatal or non-fatal heart attacks, the need for heart surgery, and effects on cholesterol and blood glucose. A total of 23 trials including 1,075 patients were assessed. Study length ranged from 2 weeks to 8 months. A total of 18 trials reported triglyceride data, and overall triglycerides decreased by 40 milligrams/deciliter (mg/dl) versus the comparison groups. Sixteen trials reported LDL cholesterol (so-called "bad" cholesterol) data, and LDL increased significantly by 4 mg/dl versus the comparison groups, but not in the studies where the triglyceride levels were high. There was no statistically significant effect on HDL cholesterol (so-called "good" cholesterol), fasting glucose, or A1C (a measure of blood glucose over 3 months). The authors noted the need for studies that are long enough to determine the effects of taking fish oil supplements on heart attacks or stroke.

- A recent report by the Agency for Health Care Research and Quality reviewed studies that assessed omega-3 fatty acids in a variety of medical conditions, including diabetes. The final report on the 18 studies in patients with diabetes indicated that omega-3 fatty acids lowered triglycerides compared with a placebo but did not affect total, HDL, or LDL cholesterol and did not affect fasting glucose or A1C levels. The report recommended that trials of omega-3 fatty acids should assess how much of the nutrient is being consumed through food and that studies should quantify the source and specific omega-3 acids in the supplements used during the trials.

- There have been two other analyses noting that fish oil use in diabetes decreases triglycerides by roughly 50 mg/dl without adversely affecting A1C.

## SIDE EFFECTS AND DRUG INTERACTIONS

Adverse effects of fish oil include a fishy aftertaste, belching, bad breath, heartburn, nausea, and loose stools. Doses higher than 3 g daily may excessively inhibit blood clotting.

People with fish allergies should be cautious about taking fish oil and should consult their physician before taking a supplement. Certain fish, such as shark, mackerel, and swordfish, may contain high levels of mercury, and fish from polluted waters may contain unacceptable levels of polychlorinated biphenyls (PCBs). Pregnant women should be cautious about consuming these fish because of the possibility of high mercury levels or PCBs passing to the baby.

Fish oil doses higher than 3 g daily are associated with increased blood glucose. There is also some concern that LDL cholesterol concentrations may increase with higher doses, although these LDL particles may not be the most dangerous type.

Fish oil may increase the effectiveness of medications that treat high blood pressure, cholesterol, diabetes, and blood clotting. However, consuming very high doses of more than 10 g daily may actually increase the risk of certain types of stroke.

Taking estrogen-containing oral contraceptives may counteract the triglyceride-lowering benefit of fish oil.

Other drug interactions include decreasing the elevated blood pressure effects of cyclosporine and enhancing the benefits of retinoids such as etretinate.

# GAMMA-LINOLENIC ACID

G amma-linolenic acid is an essential fatty acid, which means that we need to get it from our food instead of making it in our bodies. Essential fatty acids come in two main forms: omega-3 and omega-6. Gamma-linolenic acid is an omega-6 fatty acid, while fish oil is an omega-3 fatty acid (discussed previously).

The best sources of gamma-linolenic acid are evening primrose oil, black currant seed oil, and borage oil. The main source is evening primrose oil, which is extracted from a North American native plant evening primrose. This wildflower is a yellow annual or biennial that grows from 3 to 10 feet tall. The dry pod, or fruit, has many small seeds, which contain gamma-linolenic acid.

Gamma-linolenic acid is used as a nutritional supplement or as an ingredient in food products in many countries. It has been used to treat elevated lipids, infections, premenstrual syndrome, eczema, rheumatoid arthritis, and other illnesses.

## USES

People with diabetes use dietary supplements containing gamma-linolenic acid to treat peripheral neuropathy, a form of nerve damage. It is thought to improve problematic membrane structure, impulse conduction, and nerve blood flow.

Gamma-linolenic acid is not used to treat blood glucose. However, in one study of gamma-linolenic acid, some patients saw improvements in A1C, a measure of average blood glucose over 3 months. Some sources have stated that it may take several months to see results with gamma-linolenic acid.

Gamma-linolenic acid is relatively benign, and research on its use for neuropathy looks promising. Nevertheless, a definitive role for gamma-linolenic acid in treating neuropathy is unknown.

## Dose

A typical dose to treat neuropathy is 360–480 milligrams (mg) daily.

## Studies

Clinical trials of gamma-linolenic acid for neuropathy have shown mixed results.

- A well-designed study (randomized, double-blind, placebo-controlled) of 22 patients with type 1 or type 2 diabetes evaluated the effects of gamma-linolenic acid on peripheral neuropathy over 6 months. Twelve patients received 360 mg daily of gamma-linolenic acid, and 10 patients received a placebo (dummy pill). At the end of 6 months, there were improvements in neuropathy symptom scores, as well as in other parameters. A1C declined from 9.1 to 8.7%, but the change was not significant.

- In another well-designed study, 111 patients with type 1 or type 2 diabetes received either 480 mg gamma-linolenic acid or a placebo for 1 year. Patients who took gamma-linolenic acid had significant improvements in 13 of 16 parameters of nerve function. A1C did not improve, but an interesting finding was that patients who had a lower A1C responded better to gamma-linolenic acid.

- Another study evaluated the impact of gamma-linolenic acid on vibration sensation and different parameters of neuropathy. The well-designed study (randomized, double-blind, placebo-controlled) evaluated 51 patients with type 1 or type 2 diabetes and neuropathy. For 1 year, they received 480 mg gamma-linolenic acid daily or a placebo. In this study, gamma-linolenic acid did not improve the symptoms of neuropathy.

## SIDE EFFECTS AND DRUG INTERACTIONS

Most side effects of gamma-linolenic acid are mild and include headache and gastrointestinal discomfort such as bloating and loose stools. There are also reports of prolonged bleeding time and seizures.

In theory, gamma-linolenic acid, when combined with blood-thinning medications or dietary supplements, could increase bleeding. Gamma-linolenic acid should also not be combined with medications called phenothiazines (used in psychiatry), because together these medications may lower the threshold for seizures.

# GARLIC
## *Allium sativum*

Highly valued in ancient Egypt and ancient Chinese medicine, garlic has a rich history of medicinal use. Garlic has also been used in cooking for thousands of years. Its scientific name, Allium, is derived from the Celtic word *all,* which means burning. Garlic is a perennial plant with an odiferous bulb and a flowering stem that reaches 2–3 feet in height. The plant bears pinkish-purplish flowers that bloom from midsummer to September.

The bulb of the garlic plant is used in medicine. Throughout the ages, garlic has been used for a variety of things, from warding off evil spirits to preventing cancer, killing bacteria, and treating high blood pressure and high cholesterol.

### USES

Today, garlic is commonly used for cardiovascular disease and other complications related to diabetes. Some references have reported that garlic can reduce blood glucose in animals and humans, but studies do not support this use. In the laboratory, some research has shown that garlic may help repair damaged blood vessels related to diabetes.

Garlic has shown only modest benefits for treating high blood fats or lipids. Therefore, most people with diabetes will need more aggressive medication for treating lipids than garlic alone. The same is true for treating high blood pressure.

## DOSE

For fresh garlic, the dose is one clove daily. In studies, scientists have used dried garlic powder preparations standardized to 1.3% alliin content. Dried garlic preparations should be enteric coated to prevent breakdown by stomach acids. Scientists have used 600–1,200 milligrams (mg) daily of garlic extract in divided doses to treat high cholesterol and blood pressure.

## STUDIES

- An analysis of 13 well-designed studies (randomized, double-blind, placebo-controlled) found that garlic reduced total cholesterol more effectively than a placebo (dummy pill). Interestingly, the studies with the best design showed little or no difference between garlic and a placebo.

- Another analysis of garlic studies examined the supplement's effect on risk factors for cardiovascular disease. The analysis found that after 2–4 months, many studies saw improvements in cholesterol and other lipids. However, at 6 months, the improvements were not maintained.

- Another study evaluated garlic in 70 patients with type 2 diabetes who had just been diagnosed with elevated lipids. Total cholesterol decreased by 28 milligrams/deciliter (mg/dl), LDL cholesterol decreased by 30 mg/dl, and HDL cholesterol increased by 3.35 mg/dl in the garlic group. Blood fats called triglycerides did not decrease.

However, in this trial the patients were studied for only 12 weeks, so the long-term benefits were unknown.

- A separate analysis of eight garlic studies evaluated the effect of garlic on mildly high blood pressure. Results indicated a modest decrease in systolic blood pressure and diastolic blood pressure compared with a placebo. However, only three of the trials were conducted in patients who had high blood pressure. Three of the trials showed a significant reduction in systolic pressure, and four showed a significant reduction in diastolic pressure.

- Another, larger analysis evaluated garlic's effect on blood pressure in 23 different studies. Systolic blood pressure was significantly reduced in only one study, and diastolic blood pressure was significantly reduced in three studies. Twelve studies evaluated blood glucose lowering. Only one showed a significant decrease, but it was in patients without diabetes. Therefore, the analysis indicated a small, short-term benefit of garlic on lipids, an insignificant effect on blood pressure, and no significant decline in glucose in subjects with diabetes.

## SIDE EFFECTS AND DRUG INTERACTIONS

Side effects of garlic include bad breath, mouth and gastro-intestinal burning or irritation, heartburn, flatulence, allergic reactions, and, rarely, topical lesions and burns. There are reports of spontaneous bleeding reactions and post-surgery bleeding associated with garlic use.

Bleeding problems may occur if you take blood-thinning medications such as warfarin or aspirin or supplements such as ginkgo, ginger, or feverfew. If you plan to undergo surgery, you should stop using garlic.

Garlic may interfere with the effectiveness of medications such as oral contraceptives, cyclosporine, protease inhibitors, calcium-channel blockers, certain statins, certain HIV drugs, certain anticonvulsants, certain antibiotics (such as erythromycin), and drugs that are involved in certain metabolic pathways. Garlic oil may also increase the concentration of alcohol and acetaminophen (Tylenol).

# GINKGO
## *Gingko biloba*

Gingko biloba, also known as the maidenhair tree or ginkgo, has a unique history. It is one of the world's oldest living tree species, dating back over 200 million years to Permian period fossils. It is the lone survivor of the family Ginkgoaceae. The trees, which can grow to 125 feet, have a bi-lobed, fan-shaped leaf. The ginkgo species is dioecious. Male trees that are over 20 years old produce spring blossoms, while adult female trees bear a fruit that falls in autumn. The inner seed is edible and is sold in Asian markets. The ginkgo tree lives a long time, some trees as long as 1,000 years. Extracts from dried leaves of younger trees are used in dietary supplements. Ginkgo is one of the most commonly used supplements in Germany, and it is widely used for Alzheimer's disease and dementia.

### USES

Ginkgo is probably best known for its potential to improve memory and thinking. The supplement has a wide range of uses and has gained prominence not only for treatment of Alzheimer's disease, but for peripheral arterial disease (problems with blood flow to the feet and legs), antidepressant-induced sexual problems, hand and foot swelling from cold exposure, vertigo and tinnitus, altitude sickness, and asthma. Ginkgo may help with visual problems by increasing blood flow, and it may benefit glaucoma and macular degeneration.

In diabetes, gingko may be useful for peripheral circulatory problems such as intermittent claudication and for eye disease such as retinopathy. The active ingredients are thought to inhibit blood clotting, improve circulation, and scavenge for free radicals. Ginkgo's role in lowering blood glucose and improving insulin resistance is unknown. Scientists are currently studying its effect on insulin resistance.

## Dose

Doses of gingko biloba vary: 120–240 milligrams (mg) daily for dementia, 120–160 daily for peripheral vascular disease, and 240 mg daily for retinopathy. Gingko biloba is administered in divided doses, usually two or three times daily for at least 6–8 weeks.

## Studies

- The effect of ginkgo on insulin secretion has been examined in three different studies. Each study used 120 mg ginkgo daily for 3 months. The results were varied and inconclusive.

- A 3-month study was conducted in 25 patients with type 2 diabetes and retinopathy. The study evaluated 240 mg/day of a ginkgo biloba extract called EGb 761. Factors such as blood flow to the capillaries in the retina, blood viscosity, and oxygen transport efficiency improved with ginkgo. Overall, ginkgo improved retinal capillary circulation without increasing blood glucose.

Several studies have evaluated ginkgo in intermittent claudication—muscle pain during exercise—and found that ginkgo may increase pain-free walking distance.

- A well-designed, 24-week study examined 111 patients who were initially able to walk only a short distance without pain. Those who took 120 mg/day of ginkgo were able to improve their pain-free walking distance by 40%, compared with 20% for the placebo group. Patients who took ginkgo were also able to walk longer distances and walk farther without pain.

- An analysis of eight studies of gingko in intermittent claudication reported an increase in pain-free walking distance. Patients were able to walk an average of 37 yards longer when taking ginkgo.

- Another analysis of nine studies with good study design (double-blind, placebo-controlled) was also done. The trials evaluated 619 people taking 120–160 mg/day for 6 to 24 weeks. Results favored the ginkgo group.

## SIDE EFFECTS AND DRUG INTERACTIONS

A small number of patients have experienced gastrointestinal problems. Patients have also reported headaches during the first few days of taking ginkgo. Exposure to the fruit pulp may result in skin rashes, since the ginkgo fruit is somewhat similar to poison ivy and can cause allergies. Eating the seed may result in seizures, due to certain toxins. In addition, ginkgo should not be taken with medications that lower a person's threshold for seizures.

Some of the most worrisome effects have been bleeding reactions in the brain and the eyes. A recent review of case reports concluded that there may be a causal association of increased bleeding with ginkgo use and that further study is warranted.

The main drug interaction is the potential for bleeding when combined with blood-thinning drugs, such as warfarin, aspirin, or Cox-2 inhibitors such as celecoxib (Celebrex), or dietary supplements such as ginger, garlic, and feverfew.

One report indicated that a patient with dementia who took ginkgo and the antidepressant trazodone went into a coma. Also, an interaction involving alprazolam (Xanax) serum concentrations has been reported. The ginkgo lowered the levels of this medication in the blood by 17%.

Emerging evidence has shown that ginkgo may also *increase* the blood levels of many drugs, but the effects may be variable. Therefore, it is important for your doctor to measure the blood levels of medications you may be taking, such as certain psychiatric medicines, some cardiac medications, and warfarin. In addition, ginkgo may change the effects of the sulfonylureas glipizide and glyburide.

Since ginkgo may affect insulin, you should monitor your blood glucose closely. As with any supplement, tell your doctor if you are taking or are planning to take ginkgo.

# GINSENG
*Panax ginseng* and
*Panax quinquefolius*

Ginseng is a leafy, green plant that belongs to the genus Panax. It grows in eastern Asia and parts of the Northern hemisphere. The root of the ginseng plant has been used in medicine for centuries. Today it can be found in a variety of forms: fresh or dried roots, extracts, and as an ingredient in cosmetics, teas, and sodas.

Asian ginseng and American ginseng are the most popular forms and are also the forms used for diabetes.

Ginseng products have garnered attention for their misleading labels. One study found that the amount of ginseng stated on labels did not reflect what was contained in the bottles; the actual ginseng content was between 12 and 137% of what was indicated on the bottle. Other times, ginseng products have contained other dietary supplements or even prescription medications.

## USES

Both Asian and American ginsengs are used to treat type 2 diabetes. Although it is unknown how ginseng may benefit diabetes, animal research has shown that it may decrease the rate of carbohydrate absorption, increase glucose transport and uptake, and improve insulin secretion. American ginseng may help decrease blood glucose levels after meals. In one study, a type of Asian ginseng called Korean red ginseng improved erectile dysfunction, a common problem for men with diabetes.

Both ginseng species are used as an "adaptogen," so called because they purportedly help the body to deal with stress and to increase energy. Both species are also used in cosmetics and as flavoring ingredients. Although both Asian and American ginseng have been used as sports performance enhancers to help improve physical and athletic stamina, studies do not support this use. Asian ginseng has been used to enhance thinking and memory, to prevent cold or flu, and to prevent cancer.

## DOSE

The dose of Asian ginseng is 200 milligrams (mg) daily. The dose of American ginseng is 3 grams (g) right before or up to 2 hours before a meal.

## STUDIES

Ginseng has been studied for physical performance or cognitive function as well as immune system effects but has also been evaluated for diabetes.

- In a study of Asian ginseng, 36 newly diagnosed patients with type 2 diabetes received 100 mg ginseng, 200 mg ginseng, or a placebo (dummy pill) daily. At the end of the 8-week study, fasting glucose for the three groups was 149 milligrams/deciliter (mg/dl), 139 mg/dl, and 133 mg/dl, respectively. The average A1C levels (a measure of average blood glucose over 3 months) at the end of the study were 6.5%, 6.5%, and 6%, respectively, for the three groups. One problem with the study is that scientists did not report fasting glucose or A1C in patients at the beginning of the study. The impact of this study is unclear since such a good A1C was obtained in the placebo group.

- In a separate, small study, American ginseng was studied in people with and without type 2 diabetes. Scientists evaluated whether 3 g ginseng or a placebo affected blood glucose in patients after meals. In this study, a meal was simulated by a 25-g oral glucose tolerance test. In patients with diabetes, ginseng decreased blood glucose whether the herb was taken 40 minutes before or right before a meal. In patients without diabetes, ginseng decreased blood glucose only when taken right before a meal.

- The same group of researchers tried the same and higher doses of American ginseng: 3, 6, or 9 g of ginseng versus a placebo. Glucose decreased in all groups, and there were no differences among the 3-, 6-, and 9-g doses of ginseng.

## SIDE EFFECTS AND DRUG INTERACTIONS

The most common side effects are insomnia and restlessness, although some people may experience anxiety, headache, and increased blood pressure or heart rate. It should not be used by children or by pregnant or lactating women. Ginseng may be safe if taken for 3 months or less.

There are many potential drug interactions, so this product should be used with caution when taking other medications. For this reason, always tell your doctor if you are taking or are planning to take ginseng.

Ginseng may cause low blood glucose when combined with diabetes medications such as insulin or sulfonylureas. Ginseng may also increase the effectiveness of estrogen medications, analgesics, and some antidepressants.

Alternately, ginseng may interfere with the effectiveness of other mediations. It has been shown to decrease the effectiveness of the blood-thinning medication warfarin—and protection against blood clots is lost. Ginseng decreases the effects of diuretics and blood pressure medications. In combination with certain antidepressants, ginseng has resulted in mania.

# GLUCOMANNAN
## *Amorphophallus konjac*

G lucomannan has been a popular medicine and food for thousands of years in Asia. The glucomannan plant grows in Indonesia and Japan, and its plant tubers yield a chemical known as konjac mannan. The chemical is used to make konjac powder or flour, which can then be molded into noodles, rubbery jelly, and other foods.

## USES

Glucomannan is used for weight loss, high cholesterol, and diabetes. It is also used as a laxative. It contains soluble fiber that may delay glucose absorption and decrease cholesterol absorption. Glucomannan is now thought to be helpful for those who are insulin resistant, but who do not yet have diabetes, by improving insulin resistance when added to carbohydrate-containing foods. In general, people can safely eat glucomannan as food, but should be careful about taking glucomannan in tablet form due to choking hazards. Therefore, glucomannan should be consumed in a powder or capsule form.

## DOSE

Doses for diabetes and high cholesterol range from 3.6 to 10.6 grams (g) daily.

## Studies

There have been a variety of studies using glucomannan in people with diabetes. Most have involved a small number of patients.

- A study examined glucomannan in 11 patients receiving treatment for type 2 diabetes, high cholesterol, and high blood pressure. The patients were initially placed on the National Cholesterol Education Program (NCEP) Step-2 diet that limited cholesterol and saturated fat intake for 8 weeks. After the diet treatment phase, patients were randomized for 3 weeks to a placebo (dummy pill) or a treatment consisting of konjac biscuits eaten three times a day to provide 0.7 g konjac per 100 calories eaten. At the end of 3 weeks, patients had a 2-week washout and were then crossed over to the other treatment group. Fasting glucose decreased significantly from 173 to 154 milligrams/deciliter (mg/dl) in the konjac group, whereas it decreased by 1.5% from 167 mg/dl in the placebo group, a non-significant amount. Total cholesterol decreased in both the treatment and the placebo group, by 16% and 5% respectively. LDL cholesterol decreased significantly from 150 to 113 mg/dl in the glucomannan group and from 137 to 130 mg/dl in the placebo group. Systolic pressure decreased significantly by 5.5% in the glucomannan group and increased by 1.4% in the placebo group. There were no differences in diastolic blood pressure.

- A separate, well-designed study (randomized, double-blind, placebo-controlled) was done in 22 patients with type 2 diabetes and high cholesterol. Patients were on oral diabetes medications but not on cholesterol medications. The patients followed an NCEP diet for 2 months and were then randomized to a placebo or glucomannan. After

28 days, they were crossed over to the other group without a washout. The dose used was lower than in the previous study, 0.24 grams glucomannan per 100 calories eaten. LDL cholesterol decreased significantly in the glucomannan group from 154 to 138 mg/dl while it increased from 150 to 165 mg/dl in the placebo group. HDL cholesterol (so-called "good" cholesterol) increased significantly from 44 to 46 mg/dl in the glucomannan group. Fasting glucose declined significantly in the glucomannan group from 169 to 148 mg/dl; in the placebo group, it increased from 157 to 173 mg/dl. Two-hour post-meal glucose also declined by 30 mg/dl in the glucomannan group.

## SIDE EFFECTS AND DRUG INTERACTIONS

The most dangerous adverse effect is choking, which has been reported with the tablet form but not with powders or capsules. Glucomannan may cause upset stomach and may add to the effectiveness of diabetes and cholesterol-lowering medications. It should not be taken at the same time as oil-soluble vitamins such as A, D, E, and K.

# GUAR GUM
## *Cyamopsis tetragonolobus*

Guar gum is a soluble fiber that comes from the seeds of the guar plant. The plant is indigenous to tropical parts of India and Pakistan and is also grown in the southern United States. The small plant bears seed-containing pods, which are separated from the plant and used to make commercial guar gum products. Guar gum is used as a thickening agent in medications and foods and used in textile and oil-drilling industries.

## USES

In medicine, guar gum is used to treat type 1 and type 2 diabetes and high blood fats such as cholesterol and triglycerides. When combined with water, guar gum forms a viscous gel. Scientists think that guar gum may help lower blood fats by decreasing cholesterol absorption and other factors. Guar gum is thought to lower blood glucose by delaying absorption of glucose and altering the way the body digests food.

Guar gum causes a feeling of fullness and is therefore used to promote weight loss. However, studies have shown that guar gum *does not* result in weight loss. It is also used to make watery stools more solid and to decrease itchiness in people with liver disease. Scientists are studying whether guar gum tablets could be used to deliver sustained-release medications.

## Dose

In studies, scientists have used 5 grams (g) of guar gum three to four times daily with meals.

## Studies

Guar gum has been studied mostly in small numbers of patients, and there have been few long-term studies. Overall, guar gum has been shown to decrease fasting and post-meal glucose as well as lipids, but these results have generally been modest.

- In a study of 40 patients with diabetes, scientists studied the effects of two different guar gum preparations over 3 months. A1C (a measure of average blood glucose for 3 months) decreased from high values of 12.6 and 12% to 10.5 and 10.9%. Effects were modest, showing that in people with uncontrolled diabetes, guar gum makes only a small difference in blood glucose and does not lower blood glucose to target values.

- A well-designed study (randomized, double-blind, placebo-controlled) examined guar gum in 17 patients with type 1 diabetes. Patients received either 5 g granulated guar gum or a placebo (dummy pill) four times a day, before meals and as an evening snack for 6 weeks. Specifically, fasting glucose decreased significantly from 157 to 126 milligrams/deciliter (mg/dl) after 6 weeks in the guar gum group and increased from 139 to 144 mg/dl in the placebo group. A1C declined significantly from 8.3 to 7.7% in the guar gum group and nonsignificantly from 7.9 to 7.4% in the placebo group. LDL cholesterol decreased significantly in the guar gum group from 189 to 158 mg/dl and increased nonsignificantly from 163 to 166 mg/dl in the placebo group. Triglyceride and HDL cholesterol values remained unchanged in both groups.

- A separate, long-term study evaluated guar gum in 15 people with diet-treated type 2 diabetes. The patients took 5 g guar gum three times daily with meals. Patients took a placebo for 8 weeks, then guar gum for 48 weeks, then a placebo again for an additional 8 weeks. Glucose values, post-meal glucose, and lipids improved during treatment with guar gum. A1C during treatment with guar gum was 8.5%, compared with 9% during the first placebo treatment, but remained the same during the second placebo treatment period. Fasting glucose was 171 mg/dl during the first placebo treatment and 166 mg/dl during the guar gum treatment period. However, fasting glucose rose significantly during the second placebo treatment period. Mean LDL cholesterol during the first placebo period decreased from 150 to 137 mg/dl during guar gum treatment and increased to 166 mg/dl during the second placebo period. HDL and triglyceride cholesterol values remained unchanged.

## SIDE EFFECTS AND DRUG INTERACTIONS

The main adverse effects of guar gum are gastrointestinal upset, including nausea, flatulence, and diarrhea. In weight-loss products, guar gum's water-retention properties may cause the supplement to swell and obstruct the esophagus.

Using guar gum with lipid-lowering or diabetes medications could increase their effects. Also, guar gum can decrease the absorption of other medications, such as metformin, sulfonylureas, and penicillin, if taken at the same time. For these reasons, always tell your doctor if you are taking or are planning to take guar gum.

# GUGGUL
## *Commiphora mukul*

Guggul is a plant resin that comes from the mukul myrrh tree, which is mentioned in the Bible. It is commonly used in Ayurveda, an ancient practice of medicine that originated in India and that is increasingly popular in the United States. The mukul myrrh plant is a thorny shrub or small tree that grows to about 10 feet in height. The bark of the tree exudes a gummy, yellowish resin when injured, and this resin has been used in Ayurvedic medicine for thousands of years.

## USES

Guggul is used to treat acne, obesity, arthritis, and elevated blood fats such as cholesterol. Patients take guggul resin extract in pill-form by mouth.

People with diabetes take guggul for its purported benefits on cholesterol. Most of the favorable studies have been conducted in India. However, a recent study with good design conducted in the United States indicated that total and LDL cholesterol might actually increase when taking guggul. Thus, this supplement is not recommended due to conflicting evidence regarding its benefit.

# Dose

A compound called guggulipid is extracted chemically from guggul, and it contains a plant product called guggulsterones. The dose used for high cholesterol is 500–1000 mg of guggulipid (standardized to 2.5% guggulsterones). Commercial products contain guggulsterones, and the dose is 75–150 milligrams (mg) daily.

# Studies

Studies that have shown the benefits of guggul on elevated blood fats have often had problematic study design.

- One study with good design (randomized, double-blind, placebo-controlled) evaluated 64 patients for 52 weeks. The patients had a 12-week diet-stabilization period, following a 4-week observation period. Then they took 50 mg guggul or a placebo (dummy pill) twice a day for 24 weeks, followed by a 12-week washout. Total and LDL cholesterol and triglycerides declined significantly in the guggul group during treatment. Total cholesterol decreased by 25.2 milligrams/deciliter (mg/dl) in the guggul group and increased by 7.6 mg/dl in the placebo group. LDL cholesterol decreased by 16.9 mg/dl in the guggul group and increased by 4 mg/dl in the placebo group. Triglycerides decreased by 18 mg/dl in the guggul group and increased by 5.5 mg/dl in the placebo group. Blood fats then increased at the end of the washout period.

- A more recent study, however, indicates that guggul may not be as effective as previously thought. The well-designed study (randomized, double-blind, placebo-controlled) evaluated 103 patients with high cholesterol. The patients received either a placebo or two different standardized doses of guggul containing 2.5% guggulsterones: 1,000 mg three times daily (75 mg guggulsterones daily) or 2,000 mg three times daily (150 mg guggulsterone daily). After 8 weeks, the placebo group had a 5% decrease in LDL cholesterol, whereas LDL increased by 4 and 5% in the lower- and higher-dose guggul groups, respectively. HDL cholesterol decreased in both guggul groups and increased slightly in the placebo group. The increased LDL results are consistent with a recent case report of an individual who also experienced an increase—instead of a decrease—in LDL cholesterol.

## SIDE EFFECTS AND DRUG INTERACTIONS

The most commonly reported side effects are gastrointestinal, including loose stools, diarrhea, and hiccups. Headache and rash have also been reported. Pregnant women should not use guggul because of the risk of miscarriage.

The main drug interaction is the potential for bleeding when combined with blood-thinning drugs such as warfarin or aspirin, or dietary supplements such as ginger, garlic, or feverfew. Another significant drug interaction involves thyroid medications, since guggul may stimulate thyroid hormone production, meaning a doctor may have to change the dose of thyroid medications.

Guggul may also decrease the effectiveness of certain medications that people with diabetes take. These include certain statins, blood pressure medications such as the beta-blocker propranolol, calcium channel blockers such as diltiazem, angiotension-receptor blockers, and cyclosporine (a drug used to prevent organ transplant rejections). Emerging information indicates that guggul may increase the side effects of certain estrogen medications and may interfere with the benefit of tamoxifen, a drug used for breast cancer.

# GYMNEMA
## *Gymnema sylvestre*

Gymnema has been used for centuries in Ayurveda, an ancient practice of medicine that originated in India and that is increasingly popular in the United States. Gymnema is also known as *gurmar*, the "sugar destroyer," because it dulls the ability to taste sweetness. In India, gymnema has been traditionally used to treat *madhu meha*, "honey urine," or diabetes. This woody climbing plant grows in tropical forests in central and southern India. The leaves of the gymnema plant are used in medicine.

## USES

People with type 1 or type 2 diabetes use gymnema to treat blood glucose. Patients take gymnema extract in tablet form by mouth. Scientists don't know exactly how gymnema works, but they suspect that it may help the body's cells and tissues take up and use glucose. It may also improve the activity of insulin-producing cells in the pancreas.

## DOSE

Patients should use a standardized extract of gymnema. A typical dose is 400 milligrams (mg) daily, standardized to contain 24% gymnemic acids.

# STUDIES

Gymnema has been researched since the 1930s and has been studied in patients with diabetes for up to 2 years. However, target goals for A1C (a measure of average blood glucose over 3 months) and fasting glucose have not been achieved in published studies of gymnema.

- In a study of type 1 diabetes, 27 patients were given 200 mg gymnema twice a day for 6–30 months. The researchers tracked A1C, fasting blood glucose, and insulin doses. Average A1C declined from 12.8 to 9.5% after 6–8 months. After 16–18 months, the 22 patients who continued to take gymnema had a mean A1C of 9%. At the end of 26–30 months, the six patients remaining on gymnema had a further decline to 8.2%. Average fasting glucose declined from 232 to 177 milligrams/deciliter (mg/dl) after 6–8 months, 150 mg/dl after 16–18 months, and 152 mg/dl after 20–24 months. Average insulin dose decreased from 60 to 45 units/day after 6–8 months and declined further to 30 units/day after 26–30 months. A control group of 37 patients who took only insulin was also followed for 10–12 months, and these individuals had no change in blood glucose or A1C.

- In a separate study, 22 patients with type 2 diabetes took 400 mg gymnema daily for 18–20 months in addition to sulfonylureas (a class of diabetes medications). Average A1C declined from 11.9 to 8.5%, and average fasting glucose decreased from 174 to 124 mg/dl after 18–20 months. Notably, five individuals were able to stop the sulfonylurea treatment. Blood fats, called lipids, also significantly declined in this study. A control group of 25 patients on sulfonylureas plus a placebo (dummy pill) had no significant changes in A1C, fasting glucose, or lipids.

## SIDE EFFECTS AND DRUG INTERACTIONS

No adverse effects have been reported for gymnema, although in theory it may cause low blood glucose. Pregnant or lactating women, children, or elderly patients should not use gymnema because it has not been studied in these groups.

Gymnema may enhance the blood glucose-lowering effects of certain drugs used to treat diabetes. These drugs include insulin, sulfonylureas, or the nonsulfonylurea secretagoguges, such as Prandin or Starlix. As with any dietary supplement, tell your doctor if you are taking or are planning to take gymnema.

# HOLY BASIL

## *Ocimum sanctum*

Holy basil is an herb native to India and is regarded as one of the most important plants used in Ayurvedic medicine. Its Hindu name *tulsi* means "the incomparable one." Holy basil has a pleasant aroma and is available in both red and green varieties. It is planted and grows abundantly around Hindu temples, and although it is native to India, it is now widely grown throughout the world. The plant is hairy, and its multiple branches have small, tender leaves. The leaves, stems, seeds, and oil are used medicinally. Holy basil is also a common ingredient in Indian soups and stir-fry dishes.

### USES

People with type 1 or type 2 diabetes use holy basil to treat blood glucose. Researchers theorize that basil leaves may improve insulin secretion, however they have not proven this effect in rigorous studies. Holy basil is one of many herbs that are probably appropriate when taken as food, but questionable when taken as a supplement.

Primarily, people use holy basil to treat common colds, influenza, asthma, malaria, and tuberculosis. It is also used as a mosquito repellant and a topical treatment for ringworm, as well as an antidote for scorpion and snake bites. In animals, holy basil has shown analgesic (numbing) and fever-reducing properties and protection against the ulcer-producing effects of anti-inflammatory drugs such as aspirin. It is also popularly used to treat stress.

## Dose

There is no typical dose, but in one study, 2.5 grams (g) dried leaf powder were used once a day on an empty stomach.

## Studies

- Only one small study has examined holy basil in diabetes. Forty patients with type 2 diabetes were asked to stop their diabetes medications 7 days before the start of the study. All patients received an extract of holy basil leaves for a run-in period of 5 days. Then, half were randomly assigned to receive 2.5 g holy basil leaf powder, and the other half received a placebo (dummy pill) for 4 weeks. Then, patients switched treatment groups for another 4 weeks. Overall, holy basil reduced fasting blood glucose by 17.6% and post-meal blood glucose by 7.3%, and slightly decreased total cholesterol. None of the patients reported side effects.

## Side Effects and Drug Interactions

In the one study of holy basil and diabetes, patients did not report side effects. However, in animals, holy basil may decrease sperm count and thus possibly decrease fertility.

There are no reported cases of drug interactions involving holy basil. In theory, holy basil could cause low blood glucose when combined with diabetes medications such as secretagogues or insulin. Patients should also be cautious of taking holy basil with blood-thinning drugs (warfarin, aspirin, or Cox-2 inhibitors such as celecoxib) or dietary supplements (ginger, garlic, and others). Also, in theory, holy basil may interact with sedatives from the phenobarbital family (barbiturates).

# IVY GOURD
## *Coccinia indica*

Ivy gourd is an aggressive, climbing, tropical vine that spreads quickly over trees and shrubs. It grows well in India, Southeast Asia, and the Philippines. Ivy gourd has spread to Australia and has been found in Fiji, Tonga, and Hawaii. Its leaves range from 2 to 4 inches in length and have five lobes that vary from a heart to a pentagon shape. The fruit starts out green and turns red when ripe.

Ivy gourd is widely eaten as a vegetable. It contains beta-carotene and calcium and is thought to be a good source of protein and fiber. In Thailand, the young leaves and tips are blanched and prepared in stir-fry dishes, or the leaves are used in curries or for dipping chili paste. Leaves and stems are also added to soup dishes with different meats or noodles. The young leaves are boiled with porridge and then crushed and fed to children.

## USES

Ivy gourd has been classified as a medicinal herb in the traditional practice of ancient Thai medicine. It is used to treat burns, insect bites, fever, gastrointestinal complaints, and various eye infections. In addition to the whole plant, several individual parts of the plant are used in medicine, including the leaves, roots, and stems. The active ingredients are unknown, and it has not been studied well in Western medicine.

People with type 1 or type 2 diabetes use the juice of the roots and leaves to treat blood glucose. The supplement needs further study, but at this point there is limited evidence for its effectiveness in treating diabetes. Also, despite growing interest, ivy gourd is not easily found in the United States.

## DOSE

Doses have ranged from 900 milligrams (mg) of ground leaves in tablets twice daily to 6 grams (g) of dried pellets and 1 g daily of an alcoholic extract.

## STUDIES

- In a well-designed study (double-blind, randomized, placebo-controlled), scientists studied 32 patients with newly diagnosed type 2 diabetes in India. Sixteen patients received 900 mg crushed leaf powder in tablets and 16 patients received a placebo (dummy pill) twice daily for 6 weeks. In the ivy gourd group, fasting glucose decreased from 179 to 122 milligrams/deciliter (mg/dl) after 6 weeks. In the placebo group, fasting glucose decreased from 195 to 181 mg/dl after 6 weeks. In addition, a measure of blood glucose control called an oral glucose tolerance test improved in patients taking ivy gourd versus a placebo. Patients did not report any side effects.

- A separate study examined 70 patients with type 2 diabetes for 12 weeks. One group received 6-g dried pellets made from fresh ivy gourd leaves; one group received sulfonylureas (a class of diabetes medication), and one group received a placebo. The open-label design of this study (meaning the patients knew what they were taking) was not as optimal as the design of the previous study. Researchers measured fasting and post-meal glucose. Fasting glucose declined from 160 to 110 mg/dl in the ivy gourd group and from 165 to 120 mg/dl in the sulfonylurea group. Patients did not report any side effects.

- Another well-designed study (double-blind, placebo-controlled, randomized) evaluated patients with newly diagnosed type 2 diabetes. Twenty-nine patients received 1 g per day of an alcoholic extract of ivy gourd (equivalent to 15 g of the dried herb), and 30 patients received a placebo for 90 days. At the end of the study, A1C (a measure of average blood glucose over 3 months) declined significantly in the ivy gourd group from 6.7 to 6.1%. In the placebo group, A1C remained the same at 6.4% at the beginning and end of the study. Fasting glucose declined significantly in the ivy gourd group from 132 to 111 mg/dl and increased nonsignificantly in the placebo group from 125 to 133 mg/dl after 90 days. Post-meal glucose declined significantly from 183 to 149 mg/dl in the ivy gourd group and increased nonsignificantly from 155 to 167 mg/dl in the placebo group after 90 days. LDL cholesterol (so-called "bad" cholesterol) decreased significantly in the ivy gourd group as well.

## SIDE EFFECTS AND DRUG INTERACTIONS

In the limited number of studies of ivy gourd and diabetes, patients have not reported any side effects. Some patients may have an allergic rash since ivy gourd is a plant product. There have been no reported cases of drug interactions. In theory, ivy gourd may cause low blood glucose when combined with diabetes medications such as secretagogues or insulin.

# JAMBOLAN
*Eugenia jambolana* or
*Syzygium cumini*

The jambolan tree is native to India, Sri Lanka, and parts of Southeast Asia, and it now grows in South America and Florida. It grows to a height of 50–100 feet and produces edible, berry-like fruit. The fruit is about the size of a cherry and tastes somewhat acidic, although the white berry is said to taste sweeter. It is highly consumed as a tea in Brazil, but the fruit has also been used as a jelly or jam. The seed and bark are being studied in animals for glucose- and cholesterol-lowering effects.

## USES

Jambolan is included in multi-ingredient dietary supplements used to treat diabetes. There is no evidence that jambolan is beneficial to people with diabetes. However, jambolan may be safely eaten as a food.

## DOSE

Jambolan is not widely used in the United States, although in other countries the leaves are prepared as a tea and used by people with diabetes. The tea and a crushed powder form have been used in clinical studies. Jambolan can sometimes be found in multi-ingredient dietary supplements in pill form. There is no recommended dose.

# STUDIES

The two studies of jambolan and diabetes are small and have conflicting results.

- In one study with poor design, 30 patients with type 2 diabetes were given 4 grams (g) crushed jambolan powder three times a day for 3 months. The patients were compared to six patients on 250 milligrams (mg) daily of a sulfonylurea (a class of diabetes medication). Fasting blood glucose decreased significantly by 52 mg/dl after 2 months in the jambolan group, but the decrease was not significant at 3 months. However, another measure of blood glucose called an oral glucose tolerance test was significantly lower than baseline both at 2 and 3 months.

- A separate, well-designed study (randomized, double-blind, placebo-controlled) compared three groups of patients. Twenty-seven patients were randomized to the groups after a 3-month run-in period (where no treatment is given) and followed for 28 days. One group received jambolan tea plus a placebo (dummy pills) twice daily, the other group received a placebo tea plus the diabetes medication glyburide (a sulfonylurea), and the last group received a placebo tea and placebo tablets twice daily. Patients were asked to drink the tea (placebo or 2 g daily dry leaf in a teabag steeped for 5 minutes in 1 liter of water) as a water substitute. Fasting glucose increased significantly from 157 to 164 milligrams/deciliter (mg/dl) at 28 days in the jambolan group. In contrast, fasting glucose decreased from 158 to 122 mg/dl in the glyburide group.

## SIDE EFFECTS AND DRUG INTERACTIONS

No one taking jambolan has reported side effects or drug interactions. However, patients should monitor their blood glucose closely when taking jambolan. If you are taking or are considering taking jambolan, talk to your health care provider.

# MAGNESIUM

**M**agnesium is an abundant and essential nutrient in our bodies. It keeps our nervous, cardiovascular, and immune systems strong. Magnesium is also important for healthy bone growth. The National Academy of Science's Institute of Medicine has established a recommended dietary allowance for magnesium of 300–420 milligrams (mg) daily for adults, depending on age and gender. Most people can get enough magnesium by eating a wide variety of foods that include green leafy vegetables, legumes, grains, seeds, nuts, meats, coffee, and dark chocolate.

## USES

In medicine, magnesium is used as an antacid and to treat conditions such as constipation, preeclampsia, pregnancy-related leg cramps, migraine headaches, various cardiovascular diseases (including hypertension and arrhythmias), and diabetes.

People with type 2 diabetes use magnesium supplements to improve their blood glucose levels, as well as to treat complications such as nerve disease and foot ulcers. It is estimated that 25–38% of people with type 2 diabetes have low levels of magnesium. In addition, people *at risk* for type 2 diabetes take magnesium supplements because low magnesium levels are thought to play a role in developing insulin resistance. Some sources have indicated that for every 100-mg increase in magnesium consumption, the risk of type 2 diabetes is decreased by 15%. Sources of 100 mg of magnesium include four slices of whole-grain bread, 1/4 cup of nuts, or 1/2 cup of cooked squash.

However, the use of magnesium supplements in diabetes is controversial. For example, it is difficult to assess who may benefit from magnesium supplements, because there are no clear-cut guidelines about when to monitor people for magnesium deficiencies (unless you are taking certain medications or have a disease that may deplete magnesium). Magnesium-depleting medications may include certain diuretics, steroids, cyclosporine or tacrolimus (drugs used for organ transplant rejection), digoxin (used for heart failure), beta-2 agonists (used for asthma), and aminoglycoside antibiotics (used intravenously in hospitalized patients with certain serious infections). In addition, studies differ as to the benefit of magnesium supplementation and the type of magnesium, dose, and duration of treatment.

Although many persons are in favor of magnesium use because of its potential benefit, the American Diabetes Association says that more long-term studies of magnesium are needed to determine its role in treating diabetes and its complications.

## DOSE

Magnesium is available in numerous forms, such as sulfate, citrate, hydroxide, oxide, and chloride salts. The tolerable upper intake of magnesium from supplements and pharmacological agents is 350 mg daily. Higher doses may result in diarrhea.

The longest study thus far supporting magnesium supplementation was a 16-week trial in which the daily dose was 50 milliliters (ml) magnesium chloride solution (containing 50 grams [g] per 1,000 ml of solution). Use beyond 4 months has not been studied. Overall, taking magnesium supplements regularly is not recommended.

## STUDIES

Magnesium intake and the risk of type 2 diabetes have been evaluated with varying results.

- One study of over 12,000 patients assessed low magnesium levels as well as magnesium intake and the risk of diabetes. The study found there was no association between the patients' consumption of magnesium in their diet and their risk of developing type 2 diabetes. However, the scientists discovered that low levels of magnesium in the body were predictive of (meaning it may indicate) developing type 2 diabetes.

- A different study conducted food-frequency questionnaires every 2–4 years in a large group of individuals (85,060 women and 42,872 men) followed for 12 or 18 years (men and women, respectively). In this study, the investigators found that low dietary magnesium intake was correlated with increased diabetes risk.

Studies evaluating magnesium supplements in established diabetes range from showing no effect to showing potential benefit.

- A well-designed study (randomized, double-blind, placebo-controlled) in 63 patients with type 2 diabetes found benefits in taking magnesium supplements over 16 weeks. At the beginning of the study, patients had decreased magnesium levels and were taking a class of diabetes medication called sulfonylureas. Thirty-two patients received 50 ml magnesium chloride solution (50 g magnesium chloride per 1,000 ml solution) daily, and 31 took a placebo (dummy pill). After 16 weeks, the patients in the magnesium group had significant decreases in fasting glucose, from 230 to 144 milligrams/deciliter (mg/dl) and A1C (a measure of average blood glucose over 3 months) from 11.5 to 8%. Those in the placebo group also had significant declines, from 256 to 185 mg/dl and from 11.8 to 10.1%, but these values were still too high to be considered an acceptable target goal. A measure of insulin sensitivity also improved in the magnesium group.

- One study that described similar benefits was a 30-day randomized, double-blind, placebo-controlled study of 128 patients with type 2 diabetes. A total of 47.7% of the patients had low magnesium levels. Patients received 20.7 millimoles (mmol) magnesium oxide, 41.1 mmol magnesium oxide, or a placebo for 30 days. Plasma glucose increased in the magnesium groups, from 185 to 207 mg/dl in the lower-dose group and from 227 to 229 mg/dl in the higher-dose group. A1C decreased in the lower-dose group (10.2 to 9.7%) and increased in the higher-dose group (9.0 to 9.2%).

- A study that showed no change in metabolic control was done in 40 people with type 2 diabetes. The patients had low magnesium levels and were given magnesium citrate (30 mmol per day) for 3 months. A1C increased slightly, but the change was not significant (7.2 to 7.4%).

- A study on type 2 diabetes patients who needed insulin also showed no improvement. A total of 50 patients received 15 mmol per day magnesium aspartate hydrochloride or a placebo for 3 months. There was no difference in plasma glucose between the magnesium and placebo groups at the end of the study, although glucose declined slightly in the treatment group. A1C did not differ in the magnesium and placebo groups.

## SIDE EFFECTS AND DRUG INTERACTIONS

Side effects include gastrointestinal irritation, nausea, vomiting, and diarrhea. People with impaired kidney function should not take magnesium supplements because of the kidneys' inability to clear magnesium adequately.

Numerous drugs, including diuretics, digoxin, beta-2 agonists, steroids, cyclosporine, and several others may deplete magnesium. In addition, taking magnesium supplements may impair the absorption of certain drugs such as tetracycline, fluoroquinolones (Cipro), calcium supplements, and bisphosphonates (Fosamax).

Taking magnesium with calcium-channel blocker medications may lower blood pressure too much, and the person may feel dizzy. Also, high levels of magnesium may occur when taking magnesium supplements along with potassium-sparing diuretics such as spironolactone.

# MILK THISTLE
## *Silybum marianum*

**M**ilk thistle has been used for thousands of years and is mentioned in ancient Greek and Roman texts. It is a member of the aster family, which also includes daisies and other thistles. Milk thistle grows well in North America and reaches 5–10 feet in height, with large prickly, leaves that secrete a milk sap when broken. It bears pink flowers ridged with sharp spines. In Europe, milk thistle is eaten as a vegetable. The fruit, seeds, and leaves of the plants are used medicinally.

## USES

People with type 2 diabetes use milk thistle to improve their insulin resistance. However, studies have not consistently shown it to be effective, and regular use is not recommended.

Milk thistle is probably best known for treating liver-toxicity disorders, such as those due to alcoholic cirrhosis and acute and chronic viral hepatitis. Other uses include treatment of *Amanita phalloides* (a type of mushroom) poisoning and to attenuate the toxic effects of certain medications on the liver. It is used for uterine problems and the stimulation of menstrual flow. Some patients use milk thistle to reduce the possible liver toxic effects of cholesterol-lowering drugs such as simvastatin (Zocor) or glitazones such as rosiglitazone (Avandia).

# DOSE

There is no recommend dose of milk thistle for diabetes. Doses in studies have ranged from 280 to 800 milligrams (mg) daily. The typical dose for liver disease is 200 mg three times a day.

Milk thistle extract should contain 70%, or 140 mg, of silymarin, one of the active chemical ingredients. Another chemical ingredient—phosphatidylcholine—enhances absorption, meaning milk thistle preparations containing this ingredient may be dosed at only 100 mg daily. Injectable doses of milk thistle have been used in Europe.

# STUDIES

Studies evaluating milk thistle for liver disease have had serious design problems. Many studies are open-label (which means the participants know what they are taking), involve small numbers of patients, lack control groups, use different doses, lack well-defined end points (a specific pre-defined event or the target result of a trial), or involve varying liver disease severity. Several studies have evaluated the effects of milk thistle on liver disease with inconclusive results. A recent evaluation of clinical trials of patients with alcoholic liver disease or hepatitis indicated that in high-quality clinical trials, milk thistle does not have a positive impact on liver-related death rates. Also, milk thistle had no significant influence on the clinical course of patients with hepatitis or alcohol-related disease.

- Milk thistle was evaluated in a randomized, open-label trial in 60 patients with type 2 diabetes and cirrhosis. Two groups of patients on insulin were compared. One group of 30 patients received 600 mg per day silymarin, and 30 patients received a placebo (dummy pill) for 12 months. Patients taking milk thistle showed improvements in fasting blood glucose, daily blood glucose, A1C (a measure of average blood glucose over 3 months), insulin dose, and fasting insulin.

- In a separate 4-month, double-blind study, 25 people with diabetes were randomly assigned to 300 mg twice daily of silymarin seed extract, and 26 were assigned to a placebo. Silymarin was added to the diabetes medications metformin and glibenclamide (the same as glyburide, a sulfonylurea). After 4 months, fasting blood glucose declined significantly from 156 to 133 milligrams/deciliter (mg/dl) in the silymarin group and increased significantly from 167 to 188 mg/dl in the placebo group. The silymarin group had a decrease in A1C from 7.8 to 6.8% after 4 months, and the placebo group had an increase in A1C from 8.3 to 9.5%. LDL cholesterol and triglycerides also decreased significantly in the silymarin group.

## SIDE EFFECTS AND DRUG INTERACTIONS

High doses of milk thistle can cause diarrhea. Some patients have experienced intermittent episodes of severe sweating, gastrointestinal upset, and weakness that recurred after milk thistle was stopped and then restarted. Other side effects include possible allergic reactions in people who are sensitive to ragweed, chrysanthemums, marigolds, and daisies.

No known adverse interactions have been reported with milk thistle. Beneficial interactions, however, have included reduction of the toxic effects of acetaminophen (Tylenol), antipsychotics, halothane, and alcohol.

New interactions are being reported and include some reports that milk thistle may increase bleeding when combined with blood thinners and decrease the effects of estrogens. However, milk thistle itself may have some estrogenic activity and should be used with caution in women who have breast or uterine cancer. Because of emerging information regarding milk thistle's drug interactions, you should let your physician know you are taking this dietary supplement.

# NICOTINAMIDE

Nicotinamide is a form of vitamin B. It is an essential nutrient that helps manufacture fats from carbohydrates, synthesize sex hormones, and release energy in the body. Nicotinamide is found in foods such as fish, beans, yeast, bran, almonds, peanuts, wild or brown rice, whole wheat, barley, and peas.

## USES

Nicotinamide is used for a variety of conditions, including peripheral vascular disease, a vitamin-deficiency disease called pellagra, premenstrual headaches and migraines, cognitive impairment, a skin disease called bullous pemphigoid, and, in a topical form, for acne.

The vitamin is available in two major forms: nicotinic acid (niacin) and nicotinamide (niacinamide). Both forms have similar effects in low doses. In high doses, they have differing effects: nicotinic acid is used as a treatment for high cholesterol, and nicotinamide for diabetes and diabetes prevention. Nicotinamide has been studied in diabetes prevention and has been used to improve blood glucose control. It may preserve, improve, and protect insulin-producing cells in the pancreas by improving their resistance to destruction by the body's autoimmune system. Although nicotinamide may help diabetes control somewhat, the results are not definitive, and you should be aware that long-term study is still needed.

## DOSE

Nicotinamide is taken in pill-form by mouth. Doses used in some studies have been based on weight, such as 25 milligrams (mg) nicotinamide per 1 kilogram (kg) of body weight daily. For example, a patient weighing 60 kg (132 pounds) would take 1500 mg daily. In one study, the dose used was 500 mg twice a day.

## STUDIES

Nicotinamide studies in diabetes have focused on prevention and treatment. Although results have varied, the definitive European Nicotinamide Diabetes Intervention Trial (ENDIT) determined that nicotinamide *is not* effective in preventing type 1 diabetes.

- ENDIT evaluated whether regular use of nicotinamide can prevent diabetes. It was a well-designed, long-term study. The study included 549 subjects who had a first-degree family member with type 1 diabetes and who had positive islet cell antibodies, which means that the body was forming antibodies against cells in the pancreas that produce insulin. Thus, these cells were in danger of being destroyed by the body itself, putting the patients at risk for developing type 1 diabetes. Patients were given 1.2 g per meter$^2$ of modified-release nicotinamide or a placebo for 5 years. A total of 159 subjects developed diabetes; 82 were on nicotinamide, and 77 were on a placebo (dummy pill).

- A large prevention trial was conducted in high-risk children in New Zealand. Islet cell antibodies (described above) were measured in over 20,000 children. A total of

185 children had signs of being at risk for diabetes, and 173 received 500 mg of nicotinamide twice a day. Patients were followed for an average of 7 years. The incidence of diabetes was 60% lower in children given nicotinamide.

- In an analysis of 10 studies of 211 patients recently diagnosed with type 1 diabetes, scientists found that taking nicotinamide for one year improved C-peptide levels (a measure of the body's ability to produce insulin). However, after 1 year, there were no significant differences in insulin doses or A1C levels (a measure of average blood glucose over 3 months).

- A 6-month study of 18 patients with type 2 diabetes reported improved C-peptide levels in the groups receiving nicotinamide.

- Another 2-year study in 64 children recently diagnosed with type 1 diabetes found that 25 mg/kg nicotinamide daily alone or 15 mg/kg nicotinamide combined with vitamin E daily along with intensive insulin treatment preserved C-peptide levels for 2 years. There was no difference in A1C between the groups.

- The same group of researchers did a retrospective analysis and compared 25 children in whom 25 mg/kg nicotinamide daily was added to intensive insulin therapy when they were diagnosed with a group of 27 children who were only on intensive insulin therapy. After 2 years, A1C was lower in the insulin-plus-nicotinamide group than in the insulin-only group.

## SIDE EFFECTS AND DRUG INTERACTIONS

Nicotinamide is not a benign substance, and varying adverse effects and drug interactions may occur, especially with medications that may damage the liver.

Nicotinamide use may lead to skin reactions, headache, allergies, dizziness, nausea, vomiting, and diarrhea. Other side effects include blurry vision and toxic effects on the liver. Using nicotinamide means you should monitor your liver enzymes, platelet function, and blood glucose. Those with active liver disease should not take nicotinamide. It may worsen gallbladder disease, gout, peptic ulcer disease, and allergies. There is a potential for decreased insulin sensitivity and decreased first-phase insulin release. First-phase insulin release is the immediate burst or release of insulin by the pancreas in response to food intake. This physiologic response is one of the first physiologic processes that is lost when a person develops diabetes. The impact of decreased first-phase insulin release is that the body loses the ability to control glucose after meals so that post-meal glucose values rise.

Nicotinamide may increase blood levels of certain anticonvulsants, such as primidone or carbamazepine, and thus toxic effects may occur. Combination with chronic heavy alcohol use, drugs toxic to the liver, or dietary supplements (such as kava, comfrey, or pennyroyal) may damage the liver. Using nicotinamide with certain diabetes medications, such as secretagogues (such as sulfonylureas), may cause low blood glucose.

# NOPAL

*Opuntia streptacantha*

Nopal, also known as prickly pear cactus, is a succulent found in Mexico and the Southwest United States. The cactus has flat and round green "branches" covered with spines. It usually grows in colonies. Nopal has spiny fruit, which can be eaten once the spines are removed. A species of nopal called *Opuntia streptacantha Lemaire* is best known for treating blood glucose. The broiled stems of the cactus, as well as nopal extracts, are used in medicine. Some people have also used the fruit in blended shakes.

## USES

Nopal is used to treat diabetes and high cholesterol. One extract has been used to reduce the symptoms of an alcohol hangover. Men have also used nopal to reduce the symptoms of bladder fullness or urgency due to an enlarged prostate.

Nopal may help lower blood glucose if it is cooked and eaten or taken as a dietary supplement. Although some individuals may prepare a blended shake using raw nopal, the raw stems may not lower blood glucose as effectively as when cooked. Nopal contains fiber and pectin, which may decrease carbohydrate absorption. However, there have been no large, long-term studies of nopal for the treatment of diabetes.

## DOSE

A frequently quoted dose is 100–500 grams (g) daily of broiled stems. An extract containing 1,500 International Units (IU) taken prior to drinking large quantities of alcohol decreased hangover symptoms. For bladder disorders, the dose used was 500 milligrams (mg) of powdered nopal flowers three times a day. Optimal doses of extracts in supplement form have not been established to treat diabetes; therefore, you should exercise caution if taking nopal this way. As a food, however, it appears quite safe.

## STUDIES

Trials studying nopal are small and have mostly been published in Spanish, although abstracts with general overviews of the studies are available in English.

- One study was done in three groups of type 2 diabetes patients treated with diet alone or in combination with a class of diabetes medication called sulfonylureas. Patients stopped taking their diabetes medications 72 hours before taking nopal. After a 12-hour fast, one group of 16 patients received 500 g broiled nopal, a second group of 10 patients received 400 milliliters (ml) water, and a third group of 6 patients received 500 g broiled zucchini. Subjects had blood drawn 1, 2, and 3 hours after receiving the nopal, water, or zucchini. Beginning with a glucose level of 222 milligrams/deciliter (mg/dl), the nopal group had a significant decline in fasting blood glucose after 1 hour to 203 milligrams/deciliter (mg/dl), after 2 hours to 198 mg/dl, and after 3 hours to 183 mg/dl.

- Another study compared the effects of nopal in 14 patients on sulfonylureas to the effects in individuals without diabetes. Individuals in both groups received 500 g broiled nopal or 400 ml water. In the diabetes group, glucose declined after taking nopal by 21, 28, and 41 mg/dl at 1, 2, and 3 hours, respectively. Insulin concentrations also declined significantly.

## SIDE EFFECTS AND DRUG INTERACTIONS

Nopal is benign and is frequently consumed as a food. The major side effects of nopal include mild diarrhea, nausea, abdominal fullness, and increased stool volume. In one case, a patient who took nopal along with chlorpropamide (a sulfonylurea) had changes in blood glucose and insulin—although not hypoglycemia. Overall, you should tell your health care provider if you are taking or are considering taking nopal.

# PINE BARK EXTRACT
*Pinus pinaster*

Legend has it that when French explorer Jacques Cartier and his men came down with scurvy while exploring Canada in the 16th century, natives treated the men with herbal remedies from pine bark and needles. Centuries later, pine bark extract is exclusively patented and sold as Pycnogenol—the official trademark name for the product derived from the bark of the *Pinus pinaster* tree. The tree grows along the southwest shores of France. The quality of the extract is subject to French regulations and is considered chemically consistent because it is derived from specific trees that grow for a period of 30–50 years. Pycnogenol is the branded ingredient from Horphag Research and is found in hundreds of dietary supplements, including multi-vitamins and different health products.

## USES

Pine bark extract has been used for a variety of ailments, including varicose veins, coronary artery disease, and inflammatory conditions such as arthritis. It's also used to improve mental dexterity and slow the aging process. Pine bark is thought to work as an antioxidant that potently scavenges damaging free radicals in the body. It may also have a role in regenerating vitamins E and C. Pine bark has anti-inflammatory properties and may help dilate small blood vessels, as well as protect against the oxidative stress caused by ultraviolet radiation. Recently, Pycnogenol has even been found to reduce jet lag after long flights.

People with diabetes use pine bark extract to reduce blood glucose, improve erectile dysfunction, and treat eye problems such as retinopathy. Emerging evidence indicates that Pycnogenol may decrease fasting and post-meal glucose, as well as A1C (a measure of average blood glucose over 3 months). There is now some preliminary evidence for use in people with type 2 diabetes. Although there is promising evidence supporting the use of Pycnogenol, there is not enough information to recommend that patients with diabetes use this product to improve blood glucose control.

## DOSE

The daily dose used for diabetes is 100–200 milligrams (mg) Pycnogenol. Taking 300 mg versus 200 mg daily does not provide additional benefits. For retinopathy, patients in studies have taken 50 mg Pycnogenol three times a day.

## STUDIES

Although pine bark has been studied for a variety of uses, those most relevant to patients with diabetes are its effects on retinopathy and blood glucose. It has been studied short-term for a maximum of 12 weeks in diabetes; long-term studies are not available. There are also problems with study design and reporting results. Five major studies have evaluated its use for retinopathy in a total of 1,289 patients, but only one has been published in English.

- In the retinopathy study published in English, 20 patients were randomly assigned to a placebo (dummy pill) or 50 mg of Pycnogenol three times a day for 2 months. In a separate part of the study, 20 different patients with retinopathy were treated with the same dose of Pycnogenol for 2 months. In this case, the study was "open label" and scientists and the patients themselves knew Pycnogenol was being administered. Scientists measured five parameters of vision health in both groups of 20 patients. They found that some of the assessments of vision improved in those patients taking Pycnogenol. For instance, the Snellen test improved nonsignificantly in the right eye and significantly in the left eye. (The Snellen test is the test in which people are asked to read letters on a vision chart in a physician's office.) The researchers provided a subjective judgment that 53% of the patients treated with Pycnogenol received "good to very good" effectiveness, and 47% received "moderate" effectiveness.

Two studies have evaluated Pycnogenol for diabetes.

- The first study evaluated the most effective dose of Pycnogenol in 30 patients with type 2 diabetes. After a month-long lifestyle intervention that included diet and exercise, patients were given incremental doses of 50, 100, 200, and 300 mg in 3-week intervals. Every 3 weeks, scientists measured fasting glucose, post-meal glucose 2 hours after breakfast, and A1C. The scientists found that the 200 mg dose of Pycnogenol produced the most benefit in fasting and post-meal glucose. Doses up to 300 mg resulted in a continuous A1C decrease from 8 to 7.37%, and the authors reported that significance was achieved after 9–12 weeks with the 200- or 300-mg dose.

- The same group of researchers conducted a well-designed study in 77 patients with type 2 diabetes (double-blind, placebo-controlled, randomized, multi-center). Forty-three patients received a placebo, and 34 patients received 100 mg daily Pycnogenol, in addition to conventional diabetes medications for 12 weeks. The Pycnogenol group had lower plasma glucose and A1C. The researchers stated that A1C declined continuously, with a greater decline in the Pycnogenol group, but reported a significant decline only after 1 month of treatment with Pycnogenol.

## SIDE EFFECTS AND DRUG INTERACTIONS

Most side effects are benign and do not last long. These include upset stomach, dizziness, and headache. Researchers have not seen changes in vital signs, blood pressure, or electrocardiogram measurements.

So far, no drug interactions have been reported, although, in theory, Pycnogenol may disrupt the effects of immunosuppressants, such as corticosteroids, cyclosporine, or tacrolimus, because it boosts the immune system. People who have autoimmune diseases such as lupus, multiple sclerosis, or rheumatoid arthritis should also avoid pine bark extract.

# POLICOSANOL
## *Saccharum officinarum*

Policosanol is a substance that comes from the wax of sugar cane. One of the ingredients—octosanol—comes from wheat germ, alfalfa, or vegetable oil. Cuban policosanol comes in pill form and is sold in more than 40 countries for its supposed cholesterol-lowering effects.

## USES

People with diabetes take policosanol to help lower their cholesterol and treat a leg-cramping disorder called intermittent claudication. The exact mechanism for lowering cholesterol is unknown, but scientists think that policosanol may help degrade LDL cholesterol (bad cholesterol) and inhibit cholesterol production. In intermittent claudication, policosanol may inhibit blood clots.

Policosanol may be somewhat useful to people with diabetes. However, it is not as effective as statins in lowering cholesterol levels to target goals. Also, there have not been long-term studies of policosanol's effect on morbidity or mortality.

## DOSE

At this point, policosanol is a relatively benign product that may be of use in doses of 10–20 milligrams (mg) daily for high cholesterol and 20 mg daily for intermittent claudication.

# Studies

Several studies have evaluated policosanol's effect on cholesterol. Many of the studies have come from the same researchers in Cuba, using a Cuban product, and the results have been generally positive. A study in German patients failed to find the same benefit of the Cuban product used in earlier studies. In addition, a head-to-head comparison of policosonal versus a statin favored the statin's benefit on cholesterol.

- One small but well-designed study (double-blind, placebo-controlled, randomized) was done in 29 patients with type 2 diabetes and elevated blood fats, called lipids. The patients had relatively well-controlled diabetes treated with either diet or diabetes medications. After a 6-week lipid-lowering diet, patients received 5 mg policosanol twice daily or a placebo (dummy pill) for 12 weeks. In the policosanol group, LDL cholesterol (so-called "bad" cholesterol) decreased by 17%, from 211 to 165 milligrams/deciliter (mg/dl) at the end of the study. In the placebo group, LDL cholesterol increased from 191 to 213 mg/dl. Total cholesterol also decreased significantly in the policosanol group and was significantly lower than in the placebo group.

- Another study was done in 53 patients with type 2 diabetes and high lipids. Policosanol (10 mg daily) was compared with a statin called lovastatin (20 mg daily) for 12 weeks. Policosanol lowered LDL cholesterol by 20%, from 205 to 161 mg/dl. Lovastatin decreased LDL by 16%, from 203 to 176 mg/dl. Total cholesterol decreased significantly, by 14.2 and 14%, in the policosanol and lovastatin groups, respectively. HDL cholesterol (so-called "good" cholesterol) increased significantly, by 7.5%, in the policosanol group but not in the lovastatin group. Triglycerides did not change in either group.

- In a randomized, double-blind study of 69 patients, policosanol 5 mg twice daily or a placebo was given for 2 years. In the policosanol group the LDL went from a baseline of 206 to 155 mg/dl while in the placebo group LDL decreased only slightly.

- An analysis of 29 randomized, double-blind, placebo-controlled studies found there was a significant lowering of LDL cholesterol in 1,528 patients on policosanol compared with 1,406 patients on a placebo.

- One study that did not show any benefit was a well-designed study (multi-center, randomized, double-blind, placebo-controlled) of 143 German patients. The patients *did not* have diabetes. After a 6-week placebo run-in (where the participants did not receive any treatment) accompanied by dietary counseling, patients received a placebo or one of four different strengths (10, 20, 40, or 80 mg daily every evening) of policosanol for 12 weeks. LDL cholesterol decreased from 200 to 183 mg/dl in the 10-mg group, from 185 to 175 mg/dl in the 20-mg group, from 181 to 176 mg/dl in the 40-mg group, and from 186 to 173 mg/dl in the 80-mg group. These results were not significant for any of the policosanol groups or for a placebo.

- Policosanol has been used for up to 2 years for intermittent claudication, with improved treadmill walking distances. A total of 56 patients were randomized to receive 10 mg of policosanol twice daily or a placebo for up to 24 months. Walking distances on a treadmill were evaluated before treatment was started and then every 6 months. Patients who felt pain after walking at least 50 meters, but before reaching a distance of 300 meters on the treadmill, were included in the study. This was called the initial claudication distance. Patients improved from a baseline initial claudication distance of walking 126 meters to 334 meters after two years in the policosanol group, but there was no improvement in the placebo group.

## SIDE EFFECTS AND DRUG INTERACTIONS

Relatively few side effects have been reported. They include skin allergies, dizziness, stomach upset, nasal and gum bleeding, insomnia, slight weight loss, and excessive urination. No adverse effects on weight, heart rate, blood pressure, or laboratory tests have been reported.

However, people who are taking aspirin or who are on antiplatelet medications should be warned about the possibility of bleeding interactions.

# RED YEAST RICE
*Monascus purpureus Went*

Red yeast rice is mentioned in the ancient Chinese pharmacopeia, a list of medicinal drugs with information on their preparation and usage. It is used as a medicinal food to improve blood circulation and treat high cholesterol. It is also used to make rice wine and as a food preservative and coloring agent for meat and fish.

Rice is fermented with *Monascus purpureus* yeast to produce red yeast and is sold as a supplement. Red yeast rice contains compounds known as monacolins that work in the same way as statins. Monacolin K, or mevinolin, is also known as lovastatin (Mevacor). In fact, the U.S. Food and Drug Administration ordered the manufacturer of the dietary supplement Cholestin to remove its red yeast rice ingredient because it was similar to this prescription drug. Cholestin no longer contains red yeast rice, but consumers can still buy red yeast rice as a dietary supplement.

## USES

People use red yeast rice to lower their cholesterol. However, this product has not been evaluated in patients with diabetes—in the short or long term. Red yeast rice should be used with caution because of the potential for interactions with statins and many other medications.

# Dose

A typical dose is 1,200 milligrams (mg) twice daily with food. This dose contains roughly 9.6 mg statins (7.2 mg as lovastatin). A recent study used 1,800 mg twice daily, and the authors stated this was equivalent to 6 mg a day of lovastatin.

# Studies

- A randomized, double-blind, placebo-controlled trial evaluated the use of a proprietary Chinese supplement in 83 patients with high lipids (blood fats). Patients took a placebo (dummy pill) or 2.4 grams (g) daily of the product for 12 weeks. In the red yeast rice group, cholesterol decreased from 254 to 210 milligrams/deciliter (mg/dl) at the end of the study. In the placebo group, cholesterol decreased from 255 to 250 mg/dl. LDL cholesterol (so-called "bad" cholesterol) decreased from 173 to 135 mg/dl in the red yeast rice group, and from 180 to 175 mg/dl in the placebo group. Triglycerides also decreased in the red yeast rice group. There were no changes in HDL cholesterol (so-called "good" cholesterol) in either group.

- A randomized, double-blind placebo-controlled trial evaluated use of 1,800 mg (three 600 mg capsules) of red yeast rice or placebo twice daily in 62 patients for 24 weeks. All patients also enrolled in a lifestyle-change program consisting of education regarding heart disease, nutrition, exercise, and relaxation techniques for the first 12 weeks of the study. The red yeast rice group had a baseline LDL cholesterol of 163 mg/dl, and it decreased significantly to 128 mg/dl by the end of the study (24 weeks). The LDL cholesterol in the placebo decreased from 165 to 150 mg/dl. The difference between the red yeast rice group and the placebo was statistically significant. Total cholesterol also decreased significantly in the red yeast rice group from 245 to 209 mg/dl. Triglycerides also decreased and HDL cholesterol increased in the red yeast rice group but was not significantly different from the placebo group. What is notable about this study is that these patients with high cholesterol had not been able to take statins because of muscle pain and they were able to tolerate the red yeast rice for the study duration.

## SIDE EFFECTS AND DRUG INTERACTIONS

Red yeast rice may have the same side effects as other statins and may cause upset stomach and increased liver function tests, as well as allergic reactions. There was a recent case of red yeast rice causing severe liver toxicity. There are also several case reports of muscle pain in people who took red yeast rice. It has the potential to cause a serious and deadly side effect called rhabdomyolysis, in which muscles break down and are excreted in the urine. If the product is not fermented correctly, it may inadvertently contain citrinin, which may cause toxic effects to the kidneys.

There are many potential drug interactions. Taking red yeast rice with other cholesterol-lowering medications may enhance their effect and result in adverse effects, such as muscle aches.

There are many products or drugs that may increase the blood levels of red yeast rice and thus result in adverse effects. These include large quantities of grapefruit juice, certain antibiotics such as erythromycin or clarithromycin (Biaxin), some HIV drugs, and certain drugs used to treat fungal infections such as itraconazole (Sporanox) or fluconazole (Diflucan). The antidepressants nefazodone (Serzone) and fluvoxamine

(Luvox) can also increase blood levels of red yeast rice and thus produce adverse effects.

To the contrary, other substances may decrease blood levels of red yeast rice and thus decrease its cholesterol-lowering effects. These include the botanical product St. John's wort (used for depression or anxiety) and certain anticonvulsants, such as phenobarbital or phenytoin (Dilantin) or carbamazepine (Tegretol).

If combined with prescription drugs used to lower triglycerides, such as gemfibrozil (Lopid) or niacin, muscle toxicity or rhabdomyolysis may occur. If a person is taking thyroid medications (Synthroid for example), thyroid function may be affected. Red yeast rice may also lower your body's natural supply of the antioxidant CoQ10.

# ST. JOHN'S WORT
*Hypericum perforatum*

St. John's wort is a perennial with yellow flowers that grows throughout the United States, Canada, and Europe. The plant has a rich history. There are many species in the genus *Hypericum*, a name that comes from the Greek words *hyper* and *eikon*, meaning "over an apparition," since the plant was used to fend off evil spirits. The word *perforatum* is used because the translucent leaf glands resemble perforations. St. John's wort may grow up to 5 feet tall. Its bright flowers bloom in late June around the feast day of St. John, and the flowering top is used in various commercial products, including teas and tablets.

## USES

St. John's wort is one of the most popular dietary supplements and is useful for mild-to-moderate depression. The main ingredients thought to be responsible for the antidepressant activity are hypericin and hyperforin. Scientists think that these ingredients may inhibit reuptake of the neurotransmitters serotonin, norepinephrine, and dopamine.

Many people with diabetes are depressed, and they may be tempted to use "natural" products to treat their mood disorder. St. John's wort has been found to be more effective than a placebo (dummy pills) and in many cases as effective as traditional antidepressants. As with standard antidepressants, it may take several weeks to see a benefit. You should be aware that depression is a serious illness that may be successfully treated with conventional medications and behavioral therapies. If you feel you are suffering from depression, you should be evaluated and diagnosed by your doctor. Because of overall safety and efficacy concerns and the possibility of drug interactions, you should always discuss the use of St. John's wort with your doctor.

## DOSE

Doses of St. John's wort are 300–600 milligrams (mg) three times daily. Standardized extracts used in studies include 0.3% hypericin and the hyperforin-stabilized version of this extract.

## STUDIES

The studies most relevant to people with diabetes compare St. John's wort to a placebo and traditional antidepressants. Numerous studies continue to be published. Some confirm the effectiveness of St. John's wort for mild-to-moderate depression; other studies do not confirm this effect, particularly for severe depression.

- An analysis by the Cochrane Review Group evaluated 27 studies involving 2,291 patients comparing St. John's wort to a placebo or other antidepressants. Follow-up ranged from 12 to 26 weeks. In 14 studies, more patients responded to St. John's wort than to a placebo. In five studies, there was no difference in response between St. John's wort and low-dose antidepressants. Fewer side effects were reported with St. John's wort than with antidepressants.

- Another study reported greater effectiveness of St. John's wort than a placebo, but equal effectiveness when compared with the tricyclic antidepressant imipramine. St.

John's wort has been found to be equal in efficacy to the antidepressants fluoxetine (Prozac) and sertraline (Zoloft).

- A recent study reported no benefits for major depression. However, in a study that evaluated patients with severe depression, the St. John's wort group was no different from groups on the antidepressant medication sertraline or a placebo.

- Two more recent studies have reported that St. John's wort is as effective as the antidepressant medication paroxetine and more effective than fluoxetine.

## SIDE EFFECTS AND DRUG INTERACTIONS

St. John's wort can cause sensitivity to sunlight, so people taking this supplement should wear sunglasses and sunscreen. Other side effects include sleep difficulties, gastrointestinal upset, anxiety, and withdrawal-like symptoms when stopped abruptly. People should gradually taper the dosage when stopping St. John's wort. St. John's wort may also increase thyroid-stimulating hormone.

Overall, a systematic review indicated that St. John's wort is well tolerated. Four large surveillance studies that included 14,245 patients found that the rate of side effects was less than 3% and that fewer than 1% of patients quit studies because of these side effects.

You should inform your health care providers if you are taking St. John's wort, particularly because of the potential for drug interactions with medications that you may be taking as part of your diabetes management plan, such as certain statins, certain blood pressure medications, cyclosporine, digoxin, warfarin, and other important medications. Abruptly stopping St. John's wort could result in dangerously high levels of other drugs you may be taking. Also, if St. John's wort is added to some of these same drugs, levels of these drugs may fall below therapeutic levels.

# SALACIA

## *Salacia oblonga* and *Salacia reticulata*

Salacia is a woody, climbing plant that is native to India and Sri Lanka. Two species of the plant are used in medicine: *Salacia oblonga* and *Salacia reticulata*. The plant's roots and stems are used in traditional Indian medicine. Salacia has been extensively marketed in Japan as both a food and a nutritional supplement, and it is growing in popularity in the United States. Recently, a few scientific studies have indicated that Salacia may be beneficial to people with type 2 diabetes.

### USES

People use Salacia for type 2 diabetes and weight loss. It contains chemicals that may decrease post-meal glucose and thus slow the breakdown of carbohydrates. The effect is similar to the prescription medications acarbose (Precose) and miglitol (Glyset). Other chemicals in the plant may help with weight loss and affect certain enzymes that *may* benefit nerve and eye complications of diabetes.

### DOSE

One form, *Salacia reticulata*, is used as a tea. Another form, *Salacia oblonga*, has been used in doses ranging from 240 to 480 milligrams (mg) with meals. In those without diabetes, 1,000 mg have been used.

# STUDIES

- A study using Kothala Himbutu tea (containing *Salacia reticulata* and other plant products) or a placebo (dummy pill) was done in 51 patients with type 2 diabetes taking oral diabetes medications. After 3 months on Salacia or a placebo, patients were crossed over to the other group for an additional 3 months. A1C levels, a measure of average blood glucose over 3 months, were lower in the Salacia group at the end of the study than in the placebo group (6.29 versus 6.65%), and the difference was statistically significant.

- In another study (randomized, double-blind), scientists studied Salacia in 66 patients with type 2 diabetes taking oral diabetes medications. The patients received one of three treatments: a liquid meal replacement (control group), a meal replacement plus 240 mg of Salacia, or a meal replacement plus 480 mg of Salacia. Three hours later, glucose values were much lower in the Salacia groups. Specifically, the 240-mg group had a 19% reduction in glucose, and the 480-mg group had a 27% reduction. Both doses of Salacia were significantly different from the control group.

## SIDE EFFECTS AND DRUG INTERACTIONS

Side effects of Salacia include dose-related upset stomach, such as gas, belching, nausea, diarrhea, and stomach bloating. Drinking Salacia tea may cause loose stools and upset stomach. In theory, Salacia may cause low blood glucose when combined with diabetes medications such as secretagoguges or insulin. However, in the studies described above, patients taking diabetes medications did not experience episodes of low blood glucose.

# STEVIA
## *Stevia rebaudiana* Bertoni

Stevia is a food sweetener that has been used in countries such as Brazil and Japan for decades. The sweetener comes from the stevia plant—a small, shrubby perennial that bears small white flowers. It grows in Paraguay, Brazil, Central America, some Middle Eastern countries, Southeast Asia, and China. There are more than 300 species of stevia, which belongs to the family Asteraceae/Compositae.

In comparison to other sweeteners, stevia is 200 to 300 times sweeter than sugar, while aspartame, also known as Equal, is 200 times sweeter than sugar and sucralose, also known as Splenda, is 600 times sweeter than sugar. Stevia does not have any calories. In some Asian countries, stevia is used in foods such as soy sauce, pickled products, or dried seafood to diminish the salty taste.

In the United States, stevia is available as a dietary supplement and sweetener. However, there are concerns about stevia's ability to cause genetic mutations. Although stevia is widely used in Asia and many Latin American countries, the regulatory bodies in other countries have chosen not to approve stevia as a food, and some have placed limits on the amount that should be consumed.

# Uses

Stevia has been used to treat diabetes and high blood pressure and to improve heart function. However, stevia has not been studied long term in diabetes. The safety of taking stevia for long periods of time is unknown.

# Dose

Studies of stevia have used inconsistent doses, although in blood pressure studies, patients have been given doses of 750–1,500 mg a day.

# Studies

Two small studies have addressed stevia's impact on blood glucose. One was in patients with diabetes and the other was in patients without diabetes.

- One study evaluated stevia or a placebo (dummy pill) given with a test meal to 12 patients with type 2 diabetes. A1C, a measure of average blood glucose over 3 months, was 7.4%. Patients were given 1 gram (g) stevia or maize starch with the meal. Blood was drawn 30 minutes before the meal and at various times for 4 hours thereafter. Stevia significantly decreased post-meal blood glucose by 18%.

- The study in 16 subjects without diabetes found that stevia significantly decreased plasma glucose levels. However, the authors did not provide actual numbers, only a figure for their results.

Stevia has also been studied for blood pressure.

- A year-long study using 250 mg stevia three times a day in people without diabetes showed a significant improvement in systolic (14 mmHg decrease) and diastolic blood pressure (12 mmHg decrease).

- A 2-year study in 162 Chinese patients with high blood pressure, but without diabetes, also showed benefits. In this well-designed study (multi-center, randomized, double-blind, placebo-controlled), the patients took 500 mg stevioside powder or a placebo three times a day for 2 years. In the stevia group, systolic blood pressure decreased significantly from 150 to 140 mmHg at the end of the study. In the placebo group, systolic pressure increased from 149 to 150 mmHg. The difference between stevia and a placebo was significant. Diastolic pressure decreased from 95 to 89 mmHg in the stevia group, whereas diastolic pressure decreased from 96 to 95 mmHg in the placebo group. The difference between the groups was significant.

## SIDE EFFECTS AND DRUG INTERACTIONS

Side effects of stevia include nausea, bloating, dizziness, headache, weakness, and muscle pain. Some people also complain of a bitter aftertaste. In 2-year studies, patients did not experience adverse effects on their kidneys, liver, cholesterol, or electrolytes, such as sodium or potassium. In blood pressure studies lasting up to 2 years, 1,500 mg daily has been used safely without serious adverse effects other than upset stomach and other effects that quickly resolved.

Women of childbearing age, especially pregnant women, should avoid stevia because of the concern of decreased birth weight (based on animal studies) and the potential for genetic mutations. Because it belongs to the family of plants called Asteraceae/Compositae, stevia may cause allergies in people who are allergic to ragweed, marigolds, chrysanthemums, or daisies.

In animal studies, there have been reports of kidney problems, impaired reproductive activity, and some birth defects. However, sometimes very high doses of stevia are used in these studies. There is a concern that adding stevia to beverages such as colas could expose consumers to high doses of stevia, because consumers may drink large quantities.

In theory, stevia may cause low blood glucose when taken with other diabetes medications or extremely low blood pressure when taken with blood pressure medications. Since stevia may have some diuretic properties it may interact with lithium, a drug used to treat bipolar disorder, and result in elevated lithium concentrations, which may be harmful to people taking these medications.

# TEA

## *Camellia sinensis*

Next to water, tea is the most highly consumed beverage in the world. The tea plant is a member of the Theaceae family. It is an evergreen shrub or tree that may grow several feet tall, but is usually pruned to 2 to 5 feet when cultivated. The leaves are dark green with serrated edges, and the tree bears white, fragrant blossoms. Three types of tea—oolong, black, and green—are produced from the leaves of the tea plant, depending on the processing technique. Oolong tea is partially fermented, black tea is completely fermented, and green tea is not fermented. Oolong and green tea are closely related and have been used medicinally for a variety of conditions, including diabetes.

## USES

Medicinally, tea is used to prevent or treat cardiovascular disease, cancer, and obesity. It is also used to promote mental alertness, protect against solar radiation, improve dental health, and prevent aging. Green tea has been used to treat high cholesterol and high blood pressure. Tea contains polyphenols, chemicals that can have anti-inflammatory, anti-cancer, and antioxidant effects. Tea also contains caffeine, which may increase or decrease blood glucose and blood pressure.

People with diabetes may use oolong or green tea to decrease blood glucose, lower cholesterol, or lose weight. Although closely related, oolong and green tea differ in their caffeine and polyphenol content. Recent evidence indicates that regularly drinking six or more cups a day of green tea may lower your risk of developing of type 2 diabetes. Some of the ingredients in tea are thought to enhance insulin activity, which may be responsible for some of the benefit in diabetes.

## DOSE

If you wish to drink oolong or green tea, you should drink about 6 cups a day. Pregnant and lactating women should limit their tea consumption. Overall, though, you should avoid supplements containing tea.

## STUDIES

Tea has been widely studied, however it has only been studied for short periods of time.

- In one study evaluating oolong tea in type 2 diabetes, 20 individuals already taking diabetes medications were randomly assigned to drink about 6 cups of oolong tea or water daily for 1 month. Following a 2-week washout from tea consumption, patients were randomly assigned to tea or water for 1 month, followed by another 2-week washout and cross-over to the other group for 30 days. Glucose was measured after each washout and treatment period. Average glucose decreased from 229 to 162 milligrams/deciliter (mg/dl) in the tea group.

- In another study, oolong tea was given to 22 patients with type 2 diabetes. After a 2-week washout, patients were randomly assigned to drink water or 4 1/2 cups of oolong tea for 4 weeks. Patients then also had another 2-week wash-out and were crossed over to the other group for 4 weeks. A1C (a measure of average blood glucose over 3 months) decreased from 7.23 to 6.99%, and glucose decreased from 173 to 156 mg/dl in the oolong group. However, the differences were not significant. LDL cholesterol ("bad" cholesterol) decreased slightly (123 to 117 mg/dl), although the results were not significant. Total cholesterol also decreased (209 to 197 mg/dl).

- A recent 5-year observational study found that consuming 6 or more cups of green tea was associated with a decreased risk of type 2 diabetes. In this study, there was no positive benefit from oolong tea.

- Another study showed that when 240 subjects with high cholesterol were given a green tea extract for 12 weeks, total and LDL cholesterol decreased significantly (11.3% and 16.4%, respectively).

## SIDE EFFECTS AND DRUG INTERACTIONS

As a beverage, tea may not be problematic unless drunk in excessive quantities. The main adverse effects relate to caffeine toxicity, including insomnia, anxiety, restlessness, increased heart rate, and nausea. Use by pregnant women should be minimal because of unknown effects on the developing baby. Lactating women should also limit tea consumption because of problems with irritability or sleep disturbances in the infant. In weight-loss supplements (not in beverage form), there have been several cases of liver problems from products containing green tea.

Oolong and green tea may decrease the absorption of iron from foods. The aluminum content in green tea may adversely affect people with kidney problems. Adding milk (including soy milk) or creamers to tea decreases its positive effect on insulin, although adding lemon has no effect.

Tea may interfere with certain lab tests or procedures, including dipyridamole thallium tests (used to measure blood flow of arteries in the heart), and may cause false elevations in uric acid (a chemical that is increased when a person has gout) and increased vanillylmandelic acid (a metabolite of noradren-aline or norepinephrine) concentrations. For these reasons, you should tell your health care providers about your tea consump-tion if you plan to undergo any of these tests. In addition, tea may lead to worsening anxiety or worsening glaucoma due to increased eye pressure.

There are many potential drug interactions with either green or oolong tea. The caffeine content may result in toxicity when tea is combined with sympathomimetics, such as the deconges-tant Sudafed or amphetamines, or with dietary supplements that cause stimulant effects, such as ephedra and bitter orange. Other medications that may increase caffeine effects are alcoholic beverages, cimetidine (Tagamet), disulfiram (found in Antabuse, a product used to deter patients from drinking alcoholic bever-ages), oral contraceptives, estrogens, certain antibiotics such as quinolones (Cipro), or terbinafine (Lamisil, which is used for fungal infections). It may also interact with the respiratory medi-cation theophylline, the blood pressure and heart medication verapamil, the fungal infection drug fluconazole (Diflucan), and the antidepressant fluvoxamine (Luvox). In combination with monoamine oxidase (MAO) inhibitors (a class of rarely used antidepressants and some antibiotics), increased blood pressure and heart rate may occur. The caffeine content may decrease blood concentrations of clozapine (an antipsychotic) and lithium (used for some psychiatric disorders, including bipolar disorder).

Caffeine in tea may also increase the risk of bleeding when combined with blood-thinning drugs, such as warfarin, aspirin, or Cox-2 inhibitors such as celecoxib, or dietary supplements such as ginger, garlic, and feverfew. Nicotine may result in additive central nervous system effects when combined with tea, and the calming effect of certain drugs, such as pentobarbital, may be negated by tea consumption. In theory, tea may cause low blood glucose when combined with diabetes medications such as insulin or secretagogues.

# VANADIUM

Vanadium is a trace element found in several spices and foods, including black pepper, parsley, dill seeds, mushrooms, spinach, and shellfish. Some Hispanic patients identify parsley, or *perejil*, as a food that may help diabetes. Vanadium is also found in cereals, sunflower seeds, grains, wine, and beer. In 1831, a Swedish chemist named the compound *vanadis*, a nickname for the Norse goddess of beauty, youth, and luster, because the salts have beautiful colors.

## USES

Vanadium has been used for high cholesterol, heart disease, and for cancer prevention.

It has also been used for bodybuilding, but studies have not shown effectiveness for this use.

Vanadium has been used to treat type 1 and type 2 diabetes, although it has only been studied in a small number of patients for a short time. Because of its great potential for toxicity, vanadium supplementation is definitely not recommended.

## DOSE

Vanadium intake is reported to range from 6 to 18 micrograms a day, but there is no established recommended daily allowance. The estimate of tolerable upper level for adults is 1.8 milligrams (mg) daily, yet doses used in studies far exceeded this amount (100–125 mg daily). Vanadium is available as different salts: vanadyl sulfate contains 31% elemental vanadium, sodium metavanadate contains 42% elemental vanadium, and sodium orthovanadate contains 28% elemental vanadium.

## Studies

Although many people with diabetes use vanadium supplements, it has only been evaluated in a small number of people with type 1 or type 2 diabetes. It is estimated that fewer than 40 people have been involved in short-term studies.

- In a 2-week study, insulin dose decreased in patients with type 1 diabetes.

- In a separate study, six patients with type 2 diabetes were studied. Patients took a placebo (dummy pill) for 2 weeks, then 50 mg twice daily of vanadyl sulfate for 3 weeks, and a placebo again for 2 weeks. Fasting plasma glucose declined from 210 to 180 milligrams/deciliter (mg/dl). A1C (a measure of average blood glucose over 3 months) declined from 9.6 to 8.8%.

- In another study, eight patients with type 2 diabetes took 50 mg twice daily of vanadyl sulfate or a placebo for 4 weeks. Six patients continued on a placebo for an additional 4 weeks. Fasting glucose decreased significantly from 167 to 133 mg/dl in patients taking vanadium.

- In 16 patients with type 2 diabetes, vanadyl sulfate was given at three different doses (75, 150, and 300 mg daily) for 6 weeks. Fasting glucose decreased significantly only in the 300-mg group, from 167 to 144 mg/dl. A1C decreased from 7.8 to 6.8% in the 150-mg group and from 7.1 to 6.8% in the 300-mg group.

## SIDE EFFECTS AND DRUG INTERACTIONS

Side effects of vanadium include diarrhea, abdominal cramping, nausea, and flatulence that may last a few days. Some people have experienced greenish tongue discoloration as well as fatigue and small, limited changes in brain function. Serious safety issues have been raised from animal research, such as the potential for accumulation in the body and consequent toxicity. Although high doses have been used in short-term studies, prolonged use may cause other adverse consequences, such as kidney toxicity. Theoretically, it could work as a cancer *promoter*. Early reports suggested that excessive vanadium might be associated with bipolar disease. Risks of long-term use are unknown. Pregnant women should not use vanadium.

Vanadium may intensify the blood-thinning effects of certain drugs. It may also enhance both the therapeutic and adverse effects of the heart medication digoxin. In theory, it may cause low blood glucose when combined with diabetes medications.

# VIJAYASAR
## *Pterocarpus marsupium*

Vijayasar is a traditional Indian medicine that is gaining popularity in the United States. It has a long history of use by people with diabetes in India, although there is an extreme shortage of studies that evaluate its effectiveness. The supplement comes from the bark of the vijayasar tree, which is also called the Indian kino tree. It grows in central India and Sri Lanka.

## USE

People with diabetes use vijayasar to treat blood glucose. A water-solvent or ethanol extract of the bark or wood is used in medicine. Although preliminary studies indicate it has benefits, there is not enough evidence to recommend that patients use vijayasar.

## DOSE

In one study, patients were given 2–4 grams (g) daily. There is no recommended dose.

## STUDIES

Most of the studies of vijayasar have been done in animals with diabetes. There have been a few short-term studies in small numbers of patients where a slight benefit has been found with use of vijayasar.

- A 12-week study in 97 patients with newly diagnosed type 2 diabetes reported benefits with vijayasar. In the study, patients were placed on medical nutrition therapy for one month. Those patients who had fasting glucose of 120–180 mg/dl and post-meal values of 180–250 mg/dl were then treated with twice-daily doses of vijayasar at a starting dose of 2 g daily, administered half an hour before a meal. At the end of 4 weeks, patients with fasting glucose or post-meal glucose higher than target values (fasting of 120 mg/dl or higher or post-meal glucose of 180 mg/dl or higher) were treated with 3 g daily. At the end of 4 more weeks, those individuals with higher-than-target fasting or post-meal values were then treated with 4 g daily. A total of 72% of the patients achieved target fasting blood glucose, and 75% of the patients achieved target post-meal values with vijayasar. Seventy-three percent of the patients achieved the target values with the 2 g daily dose. A1C (a measure of average blood glucose over 3 months) decreased from 9.8% to 9.4 and 7% of participants achieved the study's target A1C value of 8.5% or less.

## SIDE EFFECTS AND DRUG INTERACTIONS

No side effects have been reported. In the study mentioned above, patients did not report side effects. There were also no changes in cholesterol, liver, or kidney function tests, blood counts, and electrolytes, such as sodium and potassium. In theory, low blood glucose could occur if vijayasar is used in combination with diabetes medications or dietary supplements that lower blood glucose.

# VITAMIN E

Vitamin E is an essential nutrient that is found naturally in foods such as poultry, eggs, fruits, cereal grains, vegetables, vegetable oils, and wheat germ oil. As a dietary supplement, it has enjoyed tremendous popularity for several decades. The National Health and Nutrition Examination Survey estimates that approximately 24 million people take vitamin E supplements at daily doses of 400 International Units (IU) or higher. These high doses have been associated with side effects and in one study, increased risk of death.

Vitamin E comes in several different forms. The primary form used for supplements is the alpha-tocopherol family. However, supplements containing gamma-tocopherol, the most prevalent form in a typical American diet, are becoming increasingly popular and many experts believe that this is the more beneficial form.

Vitamin E also comes in natural and synthetic forms. Both forms are found in dietary supplements, and the synthetic form is found in vitamin E–fortified foods. Experts think that synthetic vitamin E may be less beneficial than natural vitamin E. Most labels will differentiate with a "d" for the natural form and "dl" for the synthetic form of vitamin E (for example, d-alpha-tocopherol or dl-alpha-tocopherol).

# Uses

Vitamin E is used as a supplement and for treating or preventing a wide range of conditions and diseases, including aging, inflammatory skin disorders, non-cancerous breast lumps, malabsorption syndromes, cancer, Alzheimer's disease, and Parkinson's disease. It has also been used for the leg-cramping disorder intermittent claudication, nerve damage, cataracts, diabetes and its complications, as well as cardiovascular disease. Vitamin E has antioxidant properties and may help scavenge damaging free radicals in the body.

Although vitamin E was originally thought to benefit diabetes, it has not consistently shown improvement in goals such as blood glucose or A1C (a measure of average blood glucose over 3 months). There is anecdotal evidence that it may help with diabetes-related nerve damage.

The most popular use of vitamin E has been for cardiovascular disease prevention and treatment. However, several major trials have shown conflicting results, and analyses have shown there is no overall benefit. At this point, the American Heart Association does not sanction taking vitamin E supplements and instead promotes eating antioxidant-containing foods, such as grains, fruits, and vegetables.

# Dose

Recommended daily vitamin E intake for people 14 and older is 15 milligrams (mg) daily from food. This is equivalent to 22 International Units (IU) of natural vitamin E or 33 IU of synthetic vitamin E. The tolerable upper limit is 1,000 mg daily (1,500 IU of natural vitamin E or 1,100 IU of synthetic vitamin E).

# STUDIES

In diabetes, vitamin E has been shown to improve blood glucose in a few, small studies. Some studies have been positive, while others have been negative.

- In one positive study, vitamin E, given as 900 mg daily for 3 months, decreased fasting glucose, A1C, and triglycerides in 1 in 25 elderly people with type 2 diabetes.

Vitamin E is one of the most researched substances used for cardiovascular disease. However, results have been conflicting.

- In the Alpha-Tocopherol, Beta Carotene Cancer Prevention study, 29,133 male smokers without coronary heart disease were randomly assigned to 50 mg alpha-tocopherol, 20 mg beta-carotene, both, or two different placebos (dummy pills) for more than 6 years. Vitamin E use did not produce a significant change in cardiovascular disease risk, but there was a 50% increase in stroke.

- A one-and-a-half year study of 2,002 individuals with heart disease who took 800 mg alpha-tocopherol daily (later decreased to 400 mg) showed a significant decrease in the risk of heart attacks and cardiovascular death.

- The GISSI study evaluated 11,324 people who had survived a recent heart attack in a 3-year trial in which subjects were given fish oil, 300 mg vitamin E, both agents, or either of 2 placebos. Vitamin E group did not show a significant effect on death, nonfatal heart attack, or nonfatal stroke.

- In the Heart Outcomes Prevention Evaluation study, 400 IU vitamin E daily did not result in a decrease in the numbers of heart attacks, strokes, or deaths from heart disease in a trial lasting four and a half years in 9,541 subjects, including many with diabetes.

- In the famous Heart Protection Study, 20,536 individuals with coronary disease, other vascular disease, or diabetes were randomly assigned to a combination antioxidant vitamin containing 600 mg vitamin E, a statin, both agents, or 2 placebos. In the vitamin E group, there were no significant decreases in cardiovascular death or the incidence of other cardiovascular disease.

- Several analyses describing the effects of vitamin E have been performed, and the results have invariably shown there are no overall cardiovascular benefits. Not only has a lack of benefits been described, but also the possibility of great harm has emerged. A recent meta-analysis demonstrated an increased rate of death with use of vitamin E doses of more than 150 IU daily.

## SIDE EFFECTS AND DRUG INTERACTIONS

Side effects are rare, but some include upset stomach, weakness, headache, blurred vision, and rash. Adverse effects are associated with daily doses greater than 400 IU of either natural or synthetic vitamin E. Heart failure has also been associated with vitamin E use. One analysis noted that higher doses of more than 150 IU a day were associated with an increased rate of death.

High-dose vitamin E has been associated with bleeding reactions. Therefore, patients should not take high doses of vitamin E with blood-thinning drugs (such as warfarin or Coumadin) or dietary supplements that also may thin the blood. An important drug interaction has been a decrease in the beneficial effect of statins on HDL cholesterol (so-called "good" cholesterol). There are many other possible interactions with other drugs or supplements. One interaction is decreased effects of vitamin K if vitamin E is used in high doses. Many substances may affect the absorption of oil-soluble vitamins, including vitamin E, if taken at the same time. These include orlistat (the weight-loss drugs, Xenical or Alli, the latter found over the counter), mineral oil, or fibrates (used for high cholesterol such as Lopid). Some anti-convulsants may lower vitamin E levels, including phenytoin (Dilantin), carbamazepine (Tegretol), and phenobarbital. Other concerns include reducing the benefit of chemotherapy or interfering with drugs that prevent organ-transplant rejection.

# ZINC

Zinc is an essential mineral and is found naturally in foods such as red meat, poultry, seafood, dairy products, whole grains, nuts, and legumes. Interestingly, zinc binds to proteins and is absorbed as these proteins are digested. The human body is remarkably efficient at absorbing zinc. Nonetheless, vegetarians can be at risk for zinc depletion because a chemical called phytate in grains and legumes can lower zinc absorption. Zinc is available in several different forms, including zinc sulfate, zinc gluconate, and zinc combined with manganese and other nutrients. People take zinc in tablets and lozenges by mouth, and occasionally in drops, ointments or creams, and spray form.

## USES

Zinc is thought to help the immune system function optimally and is needed for appropriate cell function. Zinc is widely used for many different diseases, including pneumonia, gastric ulcers, sickle-cell disease, wound healing, Alzheimer's disease, attention deficit hyperactivity disorder, and acne, and topically for dandruff, dermatitis, psoriasis, herpes simplex eye infections, and acne. Some other popular uses include treating the common cold, macular degeneration (an eye condition associated with aging), and serious acute diarrhea in malnourished children in third world countries. It is added to some toothpaste and mouthwash products. It is also a component of intravenous feeding nutrition for burn patients.

There is some evidence that zinc supplements may benefit people with type 1 or 2 diabetes, because zinc may help the body promote insulin production and improve its action. However, more long-term study of zinc in people with diabetes is needed. Interestingly, zinc has been added as an ingredient to some older insulin formulations to help extend their action. Overall, patients should rely on a balanced diet for appropriate zinc intake, and zinc supplements should only be taken under the supervision of a doctor.

## DOSE

Recommended daily zinc intake varies depending on age and health. The upper tolerable recommended daily dose in people 19 and older is 40 milligrams (mg). For young babies, the upper level is 4 to 5 mg daily. Strict vegetarians may need as much as 50% more zinc than people on average diets. The daily dose used in one diabetes study was 30 mg.

## STUDIES

- One study evaluated zinc's role in diabetes prevention. Fifty-six obese women at risk for diabetes were given 30 mg of zinc or a placebo (dummy pill) each day for 4 weeks. The researchers monitored changes in fasting glucose, insulin concentrations, and insulin resistance. They reported there was no difference between the two groups. However, this study was only for a short period of time and only in a small number of people.

- A separate study evaluated the impact of zinc levels on heart disease in 1,050 people with type 2 diabetes. Zinc levels were measured, and the incidence of coronary heart disease death rates and heart attacks were then examined for the next 7 years. A total of 156 people died from coronary heart disease, and 254 people had a fatal or nonfatal heart attack. People with lower zinc levels had a higher risk of coronary heart disease death and other adverse cardiovascular events. The researchers speculated that zinc has antioxidant effects that protect the heart.

## SIDE EFFECTS AND DRUG INTERACTIONS

Zinc supplements may cause upset stomach, such as nausea or vomiting, and a metallic taste in the mouth. Toxic side effects may occur if you take more than 40 mg daily. At higher doses, zinc can affect copper and iron levels and result in anemia. Also, too much zinc can cause diarrhea and actually weaken—instead of boost—the immune system. It can also lower "good" cholesterol (HDL). There is some concern that zinc may worsen prostate disease.

Zinc may compete with the absorption of certain beneficial minerals, such as chromium, in the body. Also, calcium and iron supplements may decrease zinc absorption. Zinc may cause the body to absorb higher levels of manganese from certain supplements. High doses of zinc may interfere with magnesium in the body, yet high magnesium intake may decrease zinc absorption from plant sources.

Zinc may also interfere with absorption of some antibiotics, such as Cipro, or certain tetracyclines, such as Vibramycin. Some medications may decrease zinc levels, such as the ACE inhibitor lisinopril (Zestril), often taken by people with high blood pressure or kidney problems. Other medications that may decrease zinc levels include the cholesterol-lowering medication cholestyramine (Questran), steroids, such as prednisone, certain estrogens, certain acid-lowering drugs, such as Prilosec, or some anticonvulsants, such as phenytoin (Dilantin) or divalproex sodium (Depakote). You should also note that taking zinc supplements with black coffee instead of water might decrease zinc absorption by half.

# PART III
## NUTRITIONAL
## SUPPLEMENT AND
## HERB SUMMARY

# Nutritional Supplement and Herb Summary

Note: ALWAYS consult your doctor before taking dietary supplements. There are no FDA approvals for any of these products, and the optimal doses and dosage forms are not known. (In many cases, the dose provided is that found in available studies.)

| Supplement Name | Claimed Usage | Dose/Form | Study Results | Drug Interactions | Warnings |
|---|---|---|---|---|---|
| Aloe (Burn Plant, Lily of the Desert, Elephant's Gall, Sábila) | Studied in type 2, but used also by type 1. Used to move glucose into body cells and tissues. Also used to ↓ elevated triglycerides. | No recommended dose. Taken as a pill or liquid, or the inner gel from the leaf stalk is used in shakes/smoothies. Dose used in studies: 1 Tbsp aloe gel twice per day. | Available studies in small numbers of persons show it may ↓ blood glucose and cholesterol. | Potential adverse effects when used with digoxin, insulin, sulfonylureas, and anesthetics used in surgery. | Use with caution. Laxative effects. High doses may adversely affect liver and kidneys. Pregnant women should not use. Discontinue 1–2 weeks before surgery. |
| Alpha-Lipoic Acid (Thioctic Acid) | Studied in type 1 and type 2. Used for nerve damage and peripheral neuropathy. | 600–1,200 mg daily in pill form. Intravenous form used in Europe. | May ↓ oxidative stress and relieve nerve pain. No conclusive studies. Some studies show benefit, and others do not. | May ↑ effect of sulfonylureas. Antacids decrease ALA absorption—space a few hours apart. Antioxidant effect may impair benefit of chemotherapy. | No major side effects. Allergic reactions reported. May affect thyroid activity. High doses may adversely affect persons with thiamine deficiency (as in alcohol over-use). |

Legend: ↑ = increase/raise; ↓ = decrease/lower; g = grams; mg = milligrams; mcg = micrograms; ml = milliliter; Tbsp = tablespoon; tsp = teaspoon

| Supplement Name | Claimed Usage | Dose/Form | Study Results | Drug Interactions | Warnings |
|---|---|---|---|---|---|
| Banaba (Queen's Crape Myrtle, Queen's Flower, Pride of India) | Studied in type 2. Used to ↑ glucose absorption by cells. | 16–48 mg daily in studies as a soft-gel capsule. | May help ↓ blood glucose. | None reported. Use caution when used with other glucose-lowering supplements/meds. | None reported. |
| Benfotiamine (Vitamin B1, Allithiamines) | Studied in type 1 and type 2. Used to relieve effects of neuropathy, retinopathy, and nephropathy. Also used to enhance activity of enzymes involved with glucose metabolism. | 100–150 mg taken 3 times a day in pill form; sometimes combined with other B vitamins or other dietary supplements. | Shows improvement in pain relief and nerve sensation. | None reported. Some drugs ↓ thiamine levels in the body (metformin, some anticonvulsants, oral contraceptives, antibiotics, and diuretics). | People prone to allergies may develop allergy-like skin rashes. |
| Bilberry | No studies in patients with type 1 or type 2, but is used to treat type 2. Mostly used to treat vision problems (retinopathy and cataracts). | Reports that people soak berries in water and drink the juice (liquid). Leaves can be used to make teas. 20–60 g dried ripe berries daily. 160 mg bilberry extract twice daily for retinopathy. | Contains bioflavonoids. Can strengthen blood vessels and improve blood flow. | None reported. | High doses toxic in animals. If an alcohol-based extract is used, persons taking Antabuse to avoid alcohol may have a reaction consisting of gastrointestinal (GI) upset, vertigo, blurry vision, and confusion. |

Legend: ↑ = increase/raise; ↓ = decrease/lower; g = grams; mg = milligrams; mcg = micrograms; ml = milliliter; Tbsp = tablespoon; tsp = teaspoon

| Supplement Name | Claimed Usage | Dose/Form | Study Results | Drug Interactions | Warnings |
|---|---|---|---|---|---|
| Bitter Melon (Bitter Gourd, Bitter Cucumber, Karela, Ampalaya) | Studied in both type 1 and type 2. Used to ↓ blood glucose. | One small, unripe melon daily or 50–100 milliliters (ml) fresh juice drunk daily with food. Fruit and seeds, juice, or extract in tablet form. Manufacturer of a pill containing 100% dried fruit states the dose is 3 g daily. | May ↓ blood glucose in short term, but studies have shown inconsistent results. The first study with good study design actually showed a small ↑ in A1C but a very small ↓ in fasting glucose. | May cause low blood glucose when combined with sulfonylureas. | Stomach discomfort. Can cause hypoglycemic coma from teas. Young women of childbearing age and those breastfeeding should not take. Some ingredients may cause miscarriage. Persons of Mediterranean descent and some Asians should avoid due to deficiency of an enzyme needed to metabolize glucose; hemolytic anemia may result. |
| Blonde Psyllium (Plantago Psyllium, Ispaghula Husk, Psyllium) | Studied in type 2, but also used by type 1. Used to ↓ post-meal blood glucose and cholesterol. | 5.1 g, 2–3 times daily powder in water, or 3.4 g, 3 times daily to ↓ elevated cholesterol. | Yes, can ↓ post-meal blood glucose. May help statins improve cholesterol levels and relieve stomach discomfort caused by drugs like orlistat and misoprostol. | Many drug interactions due to binding and decreased absorption of medications. Includes ↓ absorption of carbamazepine (an anticonvulsant), iron supplements, and riboflavin. Beneficial interaction with statins—may have additive effects and further ↓ cholesterol. | Let your doctor know if you are taking psyllium. Allergic reactions may occur. Some forms may contain sugar and cause swallowing disorders due to esophageal obstruction. May cause gas (flatulence). |

**Legend:** ↑ = increase/raise; ↓ = decrease/lower; g = grams; mg = milligrams; mcg = micrograms; ml = milliliter; Tbsp = tablespoon; tsp = teaspoon

| Supplement Name | Claimed Usage | Dose/Form | Study Results | Drug Interactions | Warnings |
|---|---|---|---|---|---|
| Caiapo | Studied in type 2. Used to lower blood glucose and improve insulin sensitivity. Also used to ↓ weight and cholesterol. | Dose used in studies was 2–4 g daily before breakfast in pill form. | High dose (4 g) effective in ↓ A1C, post-meal glucose, cholesterol, and weight. | Theoretical possibility of ↓ in glucose if combined with insulin or sulfonylureas. | Long-term effects have not been studied in humans. Can cause gastrointestinal discomfort. |
| Chia | Studied in type 2 but also used by type 1. Used to ↓ post-meal glucose. | Dose used in studies was 37 g daily. Seeds can be sprinkled liberally on salads, soup, or yogurt. | Has been shown to significantly ↓ A1C readings and cause slight ↓ in blood pressure and cardiovascular disease markers. | None reported. | Men with pre-existing prostate cancer should avoid chia seeds due to potential ↑ in prostate cancer. May cause ↑ in triglycerides in people who already have high triglycerides. |
| Chromium Picolinate | Studied in type 1 and type 2. Used to improve blood glucose and cholesterol levels. Also used for weight loss and to reverse steroid-induced diabetes. | Young men—35 mcg daily; young women—25 mcg daily. Most common dose is 200 mcg daily, although up to 600 mcg daily have been used safely in recent studies. No upper limit for chromium intake established. | Mixed results in ↓ A1C, glucose, and cholesterol. Recent studies have found benefit when combined with biotin. | Steroids can deplete chromium. Histamine blockers, ibuprofen, and acid reducers may block absorption of chromium. Vitamin C may ↑ absorption. Taking zinc and chromium together may block absorption of both. | Can cause kidney toxicity, illness due to red blood cell breakdown, ↓ number of platelets, and liver malfunction if used in higher-than-recommended doses. |

**Legend:** ↑ = increase/raise; ↓ = decrease/lower; g = grams; mg = milligrams; mcg = micrograms; ml = milliliter; Tbsp = tablespoon; tsp = teaspoon

| Supplement Name | Claimed Usage | Dose/Form | Study Results | Drug Interactions | Warnings |
|---|---|---|---|---|---|
| Cinnamon | Studied in type 1 and type 2. Used to ↑ insulin sensitivity and ↓ cholesterol. | Doses in studies include 1, 3, and up to 6 g daily. One gram equals 1/2 tsp. Recent information indicates an aqueous extract may be the most effective form. | High doses have been effective in controlling blood glucose, especially if combined with sulfonylureas or insulin. | Known to thin blood. Do not take high doses with blood-thinning medications or supplements. | Can cause skin rashes and irritation (rare). Worsening of rosacea recently reported. |
| Coenzyme Q10 (Ubiquinone, CoQ10) | Studied in type 1 and type 2. Used to ↓ fasting blood glucose and A1C and enhance insulin production. Also used to ↓ blood pressure. | 100–200 mg daily (diabetes dose). | Variable results in studies; one study showed slight improvement in blood glucose and A1C readings. Studies in non-diabetes patients have shown ↓ blood pressure. | Coenzyme Q10 may ↓ ability of warfarin to prevent blood clots. May ↓ toxicity to the heart of the cancer drug, doxorubicin. Benefit is ↑ if combined with the antioxidant, L-carnitine. May offset ↓ CoQ10 levels caused by statin use. May see muscle toxicity if combined with the dietary supplement red yeast rice. | May cause gastrointestinal upset. |

**Legend:** ↑ = increase/raise; ↓ = decrease/lower; g = grams; mg = milligrams; mcg = micrograms; ml = milliliter; Tbsp = tablespoon; tsp = teaspoon

| Supplement Name | Claimed Usage | Dose/Form | Study Results | Drug Interactions | Warnings |
|---|---|---|---|---|---|
| Fenugreek | Studied in type 1 and type 2. Used to improve glucose carbohydrate absorption and ↓ elevated cholesterol. | Studied doses vary but include 10–15 g daily as a single dose or divided with meals or 1 g daily of a hydroalcoholic extract. | Results in studies have varied. May ↓ A1C, blood glucose, and cholesterol. | May intensify effects of blood-thinning drugs, warfarin, and herbs and result in bleeding reactions. | May cause GI upset and allergic reactions. Caution in persons with peanut allergy. May cause uterine contractions in pregnant women. |
| Fish Oil (Omega-3 Fatty Acids, N-3 Fatty Acids) | Mostly studied in persons without diabetes for cardiovascular benefit. Used in type 1 and type 2 and to prevent type 2. No direct diabetes uses. | 2–4 g daily. Must look for total amount of EPA and DHA; most supplements have only 200–400 mg, and person may need to take as many as 12–16 capsules to obtain 1–2 g a day. Common recommendation is 250–500 mg daily of EPA plus DHA. | Beneficial to cardiovascular system. Very useful to ↓ elevated triglycerides. | May ↑ effectiveness of drugs used to treat high blood pressure, cholesterol, diabetes, and blood clotting. Doses greater than 3 g per day may result in bleeding. | May cause fishy taste and heartburn. Caution in persons with fish allergies. Use reliable source to avoid high mercury concentrations. Doses greater than 10 g per day can cause strokes. |
| Gamma-Linolenic Acid | Studied in both type 1 and type 2. Used to treat nerve damage (neuropathy) and improve nerve function. | 360–480 mg per day in seed form. | Studies show mixed results. May ↑ pain-free walking distance related to intermittent claudication. | Use with blood thinners may result in bleeding. Use with phenothiazines (psychiatric med) has resulted in seizures. | Mild headache and gastrointestinal discomfort. |

**Legend:** ↑ = increase/raise; ↓ = decrease/lower; g = grams; mg = milligrams; mcg = micrograms; ml = milliliter; Tbsp = tablespoon; tsp = teaspoon

| Supplement Name | Claimed Usage | Dose/Form | Study Results | Drug Interactions | Warnings |
|---|---|---|---|---|---|
| Garlic | Studied in both type 1 and type 2. Used for blood pressure and lipids. Some folk tales state that garlic improves blood glucose. | 600–1,200 mg per day. | Variable results but generally positive effect in improving cholesterol levels. | Bleeding problems possible if taken with blood-thinning drugs or supplements. May ↓ effectiveness of oral contraceptives, cyclosporine, some HIV meds, calcium-channel blockers, some statins, some anticonvulsants, and some antibiotics. May ↑ effects of alcohol and acetaminophen (Tylenol). | Gastrointestinal upset and possible bleeding. Stop 1–2 weeks before surgery. |
| Ginkgo | Studied in type 2 for retinopathy, but used by both type 1 and type 2. Used to improve memory and reduce problems with blood flow to feet and legs (PAD), antidepressant-induced sexual problems, vertigo and tinnitus, altitude sickness, asthma, and blood flow-related visual problems. | 120–240 mg per day. | Studies examining effects on insulin secretion found inconclusive results. Major use may be to increase pain-free walking distance and to improve retinal capillary circulation. | Increased potential for bleeding when combined with blood-thinning drugs, or Cox-2 inhibitors, or the supplements ginger, garlic, and feverfew. May change the effects of glipizide and glyburide (sulfonylureas). | Exposure to ginkgo fruit pulp may cause skin rashes. Increased bleeding possible; stop 1–2 weeks before surgery. |

**Legend:** ↑ = increase/raise; ↓ = decrease/lower; g = grams; mg = milligrams; mcg = micrograms; ml = milliliter; Tbsp = tablespoon; tsp = teaspoon

| Supplement Name | Claimed Usage | Dose/Form | Study Results | Drug Interactions | Warnings |
|---|---|---|---|---|---|
| Ginseng (Asian Ginseng, American Ginseng) | Studied in type 2 but used by both type 1 and type 2. Used to ↑ energy, ↓ rate of carbohydrate absorption, ↑ glucose transport and uptake, and improve insulin secretion. | Asian ginseng: 200 mg per day. American ginseng: 3 g before a meal. | Variable results, but studies show ginseng ↓ blood glucose, and American ginseng may improve post-meal glucose. | Decreases effectiveness of blood thinners, diuretics, and BP medications. May cause hypoglycemia when used with insulin and sulfonylureas. May ↑ effects of estrogens, some analgesics, and antidepressants (may see mania emerge in bipolar patients). | Can cause insomnia, headache, restlessness, and ↑ blood pressure. Children or pregnant/ lactating women should not take ginseng. |
| Glucomannan (Konjac, Konjac Mannan) | Studied in type 2, but used by both type 1 and type 2. Used to promote weight loss and ↓ high cholesterol and glucose. | 3.6–10.6 g per day. Taken as powder or capsule. | Studies are generally positive and have shown ↓ fasting and post-meal glucose and improved cholesterol. | May ↓ absorption of oil-soluble vitamins, such as A, D, E, and K if taken at the same time. | Tablet form (but not powders or capsules) can result in choking. May cause gastrointestinal upset. |
| Guar Gum (Indian Cluster Bean) | Studied in both type 1 and type 2. Used to ↓ blood glucose by delaying absorption of glucose. Also used to ↓ cholesterol absorption and promote weight loss. | 5 g, 3–4 times a day with meals in powder form added to foods. | Studies show modest effectiveness in ↓ A1C, glucose, and lipids. | Can ↓ the absorption of medications, such as metformin, sulfonyl-ureas, and penicillin if taken at the same time. | Adverse effects include gastrointestinal upset. Water-retention properties can lead to product swelling and result in esophageal obstruction and choking hazard. |

**Legend:** ↑ = increase/raise; ↓ = decrease/lower; g = grams; mg = milligrams; mcg = micrograms; ml = milliliter; Tbsp = tablespoon; tsp = teaspoon

| Supplement Name | Claimed Usage | Dose/Form | Study Results | Drug Interactions | Warnings |
|---|---|---|---|---|---|
| Guggul (Guggulipid, Guggulu) | Not studied specifically for diabetes but taken by both type 1 and type 2. Used to help control cholesterol. | 75–150 mg per day of standardized guggulsterones taken in pill form. | Studies have shown mixed results, with some showing benefit in ↓ elevated cholesterol and others showing it actually ↑ cholesterol. | Potential for ↑ bleeding when taken with blood-thinning drugs, such as warfarin, aspirin, or certain supplements (ginger, garlic, and feverfew). May ↓ benefit of blood pressure meds, statins, and organ transplant rejection drugs. May ↑ side effects of estrogens and offset benefit of tamoxifen in cancer patients. May affect dose of thyroid supplements. | Pregnant women must not take, because of heightened risk of miscarriage. Headache, rash, and gastrointestinal upset have occurred. |
| Gymnema (Gymnema sylvestre) | Studied in both type 1 and type 2. Used to help the body take up and use blood glucose. Also used to improve function of cells in pancreas. | 400 mg per day, standardized to 24% gymnemic acids in pill form. | Older studies lack good study design but show some benefit in ↓ glucose and cholesterol. There are ongoing studies in the United States. | May cause acute hypoglycemia if combined with insulin, sulfonylureas, and non-sulfonylurea secretagogues. | Pregnant or lactating women, children, or elderly patients should not use gymnema, because it has not been studied in these populations. |

Legend: ↑ = increase/raise; ↓ = decrease/lower; g = grams; mg = milligrams; mcg = micrograms; ml = milliliter; Tbsp = tablespoon; tsp = teaspoon

| Supplement Name | Claimed Usage | Dose/Form | Study Results | Drug Interactions | Warnings |
|---|---|---|---|---|---|
| Holy Basil (Sacred Basil, Green Holy Basil, Hot Basil) | Studied only in type 2 but used by both type 1 and type 2. Used to help improve insulin secretion. | No recommended dose. In studies, 2.5 g dried leaf power was taken orally daily. | Only one study with good study design, which indicated that fasting and post-meal glucose ↓. | May cause low blood glucose when used with secretagogues or insulin. Use caution when taking with blood thinners (drugs or supplements). May also interact with phenobarbital. | In animals, there is ↓ sperm count, so question of ↓ fertility. |
| Ivy Gourd | Studied in type 2 but used by both type 1 and 2. Used to treat blood glucose. | No standard dose; used in oral form. Doses range from 900 mg of ground leaves in tablets 2 times a day to 6 g dried pellets and 1 g of an alcohol extract (15 g of the dried herb) daily. | Some well-designed studies have shown ↓ A1C, as well as fasting and post-meal glucose. Cholesterol has also ↓ in some studies. | Possibility of hypoglycemia if combined with drugs that ↓ glucose, such as insulin or secretagogues. | Possible rash, since this is a plant product. |
| Jambolan (Jambul, Jamun Beej, Java Plum, Rose Apple) | Studied in type 2 but possibly used by both type 1 and type 2. Used to ↓ glucose. | No standard dose; studies have used 4 g of crushed powder 3 times a day or 2 g daily dry leaf tea. | Small studies have shown both ↓ and ↑ fasting glucose in the short term. | No reported drug interactions. | No reported side effects. |

Legend: ↑ = increase/raise; ↓ = decrease/lower; g = grams; mg = milligrams; mcg = micrograms; ml = milliliter; Tbsp = tablespoon; tsp = teaspoon

| Supplement Name | Claimed Usage | Dose/Form | Study Results | Drug Interactions | Warnings |
|---|---|---|---|---|---|
| Magnesium | Studied in type 2 but used by both type 1 and type 2. Used to regulate blood glucose and complications, such as nerve disease and foot ulcers. Also used to prevent type 2. | No standard dose, but 50 ml solution of magnesium chloride has been used. Tolerable upper intake is 350 mg daily. | Varying results in studies. Some studies showed ↓ A1C and fasting glucose and others did not. Low levels of magnesium may point to a risk for type 2. | May impair absorption of some drugs, such as, tetracycline, fluoroquinolones, calcium supplements, and bisphosphonates. Many drugs deplete magnesium (certain diuretics, digoxin, asthma meds, organ transplant–rejection drugs). Some drugs may ↑ magnesium (spironolactone and other potassium-sparing diuretics). If taken with calcium-channel blocker medications, blood pressure may ↓. | Gastrointestinal upset, vomiting, and diarrhea. Persons with impaired kidney function should avoid, since they cannot excrete magnesium adequately. |

Legend: ↑ = increase/raise; ↓ = decrease/lower; g = grams; mg = milligrams; mcg = micrograms; ml = milliliter; Tbsp = tablespoon; tsp = teaspoon

| Supplement Name | Claimed Usage | Dose/Form | Study Results | Drug Interactions | Warnings |
|---|---|---|---|---|---|
| Milk Thistle | Studied in type 2 but may be used by both type 1 and type 2. Used to improve insulin resistance, ↓ elevated glucose, and for liver protection against toxic drugs. | Doses range from 280 to 800 mg per day, taken in pill form. A common dose is 200 mg, 3 times a day (must contain 70% silymarin). | Shown to ↓ A1C, fasting glucose, and cholesterol. | May ↑ bleeding if combined with blood thinners. May ↓ effects of estrogens. May ↓ liver toxic effects of acetaminophen and alcohol. | High doses of milk thistle can cause gastrointestinal upset and diarrhea; allergic reactions if sensitive to ragweed and daisy family. Due to estrogenic effects, women with breast or uterine cancer should not use. |
| Nicotinamide | Studied in type 1 and type 2. Used to improve blood glucose control and help peripheral vascular disease. Used to prevent diabetes and to control cholesterol. | Inconsistent dosing, but may dose based on weight: 25 mg of nicotinamide per 1 kg of body weight in pill form (for example, a 60-kg person would take 1500 mg daily). A dose of 500 mg twice daily has been used. | Variable results in studies. May improve C-peptide levels but not consistently lower A1C. Not effective to prevent type 1 diabetes. | Combination with chronic heavy alcohol use or liver toxic drugs, or dietary supplements (kava, comfrey, and pennyroyal) may damage the liver. May ↑ levels of certain anticonvulsants. | People with active liver disease should not take nicotinamide. May cause rashes, gastrointestinal upset, blurred vision, or liver damage. May worsen gall bladder disease, gout, ulcers, and allergies. |
| Nopal (Prickly Pear) | Studied in type 2 but used by both type 1 and type 2. Used to ↓ blood glucose and high cholesterol. | 100–500 g per day as broiled stems, in liquid form, or prepared as shakes/smoothies. | Small short-term studies have shown it to be effective in ↓ blood glucose. | No significant drug interactions. Nopal is benign and frequently used as a food. | Due to fiber content, may cause diarrhea. |

**Legend:** ↑ = increase/raise; ↓ = decrease/lower; g = grams; mg = milligrams; mcg = micrograms; ml = milliliter; Tbsp = tablespoon; tsp = teaspoon

| Supplement Name | Claimed Usage | Dose/Form | Study Results | Drug Interactions | Warnings |
|---|---|---|---|---|---|
| Pine Bark Extract (Pycnogenol) | Studied in type 2 but used by both type 1 and 2 to improve retinopathy | 100 to 200 mg/day in pill form. | Small studies show improved vision and ↓ A1C, fasting and post-meal glucose. | No drug interactions reported but theoretically may antagonize effects of steroids and organ transplant–rejection drugs, since pine bark extract boosts the immune system. Side effects: Minor stomach upset, dizziness, and headache. | People with immune system disorders, such as lupus, multiple sclerosis, or rheumatoid arthritis, should not take pine bark extract. |
| Policosanol | Studied in type 2 but used by both type 1 and 2 to lower cholesterol and treat leg cramps (intermittent claudication). | 10 to 20 mg/day for high cholesterol and 20 mg/day for intermittent claudication (leg cramps) in pill form. | Does ↓ high cholesterol, but not as effectively as statins. | May ↑ risk of bleeding if taken with blood thinners (aspirin or supplements or other drugs with anticoagulant effects). | May see skin allergies, dizziness, GI upset, nose and gum bleeding, insomnia, weight loss and excessive urination. |

Legend: ↑ = increase/raise; ↓ = decrease/lower; g = grams; mg = milligrams; mcg = micrograms; ml = milliliter; Tbsp = tablespoon; tsp = teaspoon

| Supplement Name | Claimed Usage | Dose/Form | Study Results | Drug Interactions | Warnings |
|---|---|---|---|---|---|
| Red Yeast Rice (Red Yeast, XueZhiKang) | Not studied in diabetes, but used by both type 1 and type 2. Used to ↓ cholesterol. | 1,200 mg to 1,800 mg twice a day with food in pill form (equivalent to approximately 6 to 7.2 mg of lovastatin). | Only a few studies, but they show ↓ LDL cholesterol and triglycerides. Contains monacolins that work the same as statins. | Many potential drug interactions due to statin content. May cause muscle cramps if taken with erythromycin, some antifungals, HIV drugs, some antidepressants, gemfibrozil, and large quantities of grapefruit juice. Taking it with other cholesterol-lowering medications may enhance their action and result in adverse effects, such as muscle aches. May ↓ body's supply of CoQ10. | Like statins, may rarely cause liver toxicity and muscle aches. If not fermented correctly, it may contain citrinin, which may cause toxic effects to the kidneys. May affect thyroid function. |
| St. John's Wort | Not studied in diabetes but used by both type 1 and type 2. Used to treat mild-to-moderate depression. | 300–600 mg three times a day in pill form. | Effective for mild depression. | Numerous drug interactions. May ↓ blood levels of many drugs (blood pressure, statins, HIV, blood thinners, oral contraceptives). | Can cause sensitivity to sunlight, sunburn, and cataracts. Do not discontinue use abruptly, and do not use without physician supervision. |

**Legend:** ↑ = increase/raise; ↓ = decrease/lower; g = grams; mg = milligrams; mcg = micrograms; ml = milliliter; Tbsp = tablespoon; tsp = teaspoon

| Supplement Name | Claimed Usage | Dose/Form | Study Results | Drug Interactions | Warnings |
|---|---|---|---|---|---|
| Salacia | Studied in type 2 but used by both type 1 and type 2. Used for weight loss. | Two forms: Salacia reticulata used as a tea. Salacia oblonga dose ranges from 240 to 480 mg with meals in pill form. | Some studies show salacia may ↓ A1C and post-meal glucose, acting similarly to an alpha glucosidase inhibitor. | May cause low blood glucose if combined with insulin or secretagoguges. | Upset stomach and diarrhea. |
| Stevia | Studied in type 2, but used in both type 1 and 2. Used as a food sweetener and sugar substitute and for high blood pressure and high glucose. | No recommended dose. For blood pressure studies, dose 750–1,500 mg per day in pill form. | Studies have shown ↓ postmeal glucose in diabetes and ↓ blood pressure in persons without diabetes. | Possible low glucose if combined with insulin or secretagoguges. Since stevia has diuretic effects, it may ↑ lithium levels. | Bitter taste, stomach upset, headache, muscle pain, and possible allergies. Birth defects in animals lead to concerns that stevia may cause genetic mutations. Long-term safety unknown. Women of childbearing age should avoid stevia. |

**Legend:** ↑ = increase/raise; ↓ = decrease/lower; g = grams; mg = milligrams; mcg = micrograms; ml = milliliter; Tbsp = tablespoon; tsp = teaspoon

| Supplement Name | Claimed Usage | Dose/Form | Study Results | Drug Interactions | Warnings |
|---|---|---|---|---|---|
| Tea (Black, Oolong, and Green) | Studied in type 2 but used in both type 1 and type 2. Oolong and green tea are used to ↓ blood glucose, cholesterol, and body weight. | Up to 6 cups per day. | Small studies have shown small decreases in A1C and glucose. Drinking green tea may lower risk of diabetes. | Many drugs ↑ caffeine effects (decongestants, contraceptives, estrogens, certain antibiotics, and antifungals). Caffeine content may ↓ levels of some psychiatric drugs, and cause ↑ bleeding if used with blood thinners. It can interfere with certain lab tests. | May cause insomnia, anxiety, and restlessness due to caffeine content. Pregnant and lactating women should limit tea consumption. |
| Vanadium | Studied in type 1 and type 2. Used to ↓ blood glucose. Also used for high cholesterol, heart disease, and cancer prevention. | No recommended dose. Estimated tolerable upper level for adults is 1.8 mg per day. Studies used very high doses. | Few short-term studies with small numbers of subjects showed ↓ blood glucose. | May intensify bleeding if combined with blood thinners. Adverse effects with heart medication digoxin. | Gastrointestinal upset and may accumulate in tissues. High potential for toxicity. Do not use. |
| Vijayasar | Studied in type 2 but used in type 1 and type 2. Used to ↓ blood glucose. | No recommended dose, but 2–4 g daily were used in a study. | Short-term studies have shown ↓ A1C, fasting, and post-meal glucose. | None reported. | None reported. |

**Legend:** ↑ = increase/raise; ↓ = decrease/lower; g = grams; mg = milligrams; mcg = micrograms; ml = milliliter; Tbsp = tablespoon; tsp = teaspoon

| Supplement Name | Claimed Usage | Dose/Form | Study Results | Drug Interactions | Warnings |
|---|---|---|---|---|---|
| Vitamin E | Studied in type 2 but used in type 1 and type 2. Essential nutrient that is used to help diabetes-related nerve damage. | Recommended dose is 15 mg daily from food for adults. Tolerable upper limit is 1,000 mg daily (1,500 IU of natural vitamin E or 1,100 IU of synthetic vitamin E). | Studies inconclusive. Studies show no benefit for cardiovascular disease. Mortality ↑ if doses greater than 150 IU daily are used. Gamma tocopherol may be a beneficial form. | High doses of vitamin E may interfere with blood-thinning drugs. May ↓ beneficial effects of statins in increasing HDL. Absorption of vitamin E ↓ if taken with orlistat, mineral oil, fibrates, or some anti-convulsants. Vitamin E may ↓ effects of chemotherapy. | Gastrointestinal upset, rash, headache, and blurred vision. Bleeding with high doses. Use with caution. |

Legend: ↑ = increase/raise; ↓ = decrease/lower; g = grams; mg = milligrams; mcg = micrograms; ml = milliliter; Tbsp = tablespoon; tsp = teaspoon

| Supplement Name | Claimed Usage | Dose/Form | Study Results | Drug Interactions | Warnings |
|---|---|---|---|---|---|
| Zinc | Studied mostly in type 2 but used by both type 1 and type 2. Used to help ↑ insulin production and action. | No recommended dose. Upper tolerable adult dose is 40 mg daily. | Studies are inconclusive, but zinc deficiency is associated with diabetes and cardiovascular disease. | Some minerals impair zinc absorption (calcium, iron, magnesium). Drinking black coffee may impair zinc absorption. May affect copper and iron levels at high doses. Zinc may cause higher absorption of manganese from certain supplements. Zinc may interfere with absorption of some antibiotics and some medications (ACE inhibitors, steroids, bile acid sequestrants, acid suppressors, some anticonvulsants) may decrease zinc levels. | Gastrointestinal upset and metallic taste. Some concern that zinc may worsen prostate disease. May weaken the immune system. |

**Legend:** ↑ = increase/raise; ↓ = decrease/lower; g = grams; mg = milligrams; mcg = micrograms; ml = milliliter; Tbsp = tablespoon; tsp = teaspoon

# INDEX

Aspirin interactions
  ginkgo, 84
  guggul, 97, 175
  holy basil, 103, 176
  policosanol, 132, 179
  tea/caffeine, 150, 182

# B

Banaba (crape myrtle), 31–32, 168

Barbiturates, 103

Basil, 101–103, 176

Benfotiamine, 33–35, 168

Beta-2 agonists, 111, 114

Bias in clinical studies, 17, 18

Bilberry, 36–38, 168

Biloba. *See* Ginkgo biloba

Bisphosphonates, 114, 177

Bitter melon, 39–42, 169

Bitter orange, 149

Blonde psyllium, 43–46, 169

Blood clotting, 38, 73

Breast feeding drug interactions
  aloe, 35
  bitter melon, 41, 169
  fenugreek, 66
  ginseng, 87, 174
  gymnema, 100, 175
  tea, 147, 148, 182

# C

Caffeine, 146–150, 182

Caiapo, 47–48, 170

Calcium channel blockers, 97, 114, 173, 177

Carbamazepine (Tegretol), 46, 121, 136, 160, 169

Cardiovascular disease, 70, 71

Cassia (cinnamon), 57–59, 171

Cataracts, 36, 37

Celecoxib (Celebrex), 84, 103, 150

Chemotherapy, 30, 35, 160, 167, 183

Chia, 49–51, 170

Chlorpropamide, 124

Cholestin, 133

Cholestyramine (Questran), 164

Chromium, 36, 52–56, 170

Cimetidine (Tagamet), 149

Cinnamon (cassia), 57–59, 171

Cipro, 114, 149, 163, 184

Clarithromycin (Biaxin), 135

Clinical studies, 13, 16–19

Clozapine, 149

Cochrane Collaboration trials, 72

Coenzyme Q10, 60–65, 136, 170, 180

Congestive heart failure, 62–63

Consumer Lab, 12

Consumers Union, 12

Corticosteriods, 128

Coumadin, 159

Cox-2 inhibitors, 84, 103, 150, 173

Crape myrtle (banaba), 31–32, 168

Cross-over studies, 19

Cyclosporine interactions
  garlic, 97, 173
  magnesium, 111, 114, 177
  pycnogenol, 128
  St. John's wort, 139, 180

# D

Dietary Supplement Health and Education Act, 9

Dietary supplements
discussing with health care providers, 6–8
evaluation of, 12–16
labeling/content, 9–11
overview, 3–5
packs, 14
recommended daily allowances, 14
regulation of, 8–9
research resources, 8

Digoxin interactions
aloe, 25, 167
magnesium, 111, 114, 177
St. John's wort, 139, 180
vanadium, 182

Diltiazem, 97

Disulfiram, 149

Diuretics, 111, 114, 177

Divalproex sodium (Depakote), 164

Double-blind studies, 17

Doxorubicin, 65, 171

Drug interactions, 5–6

# E

Echinacea, 11

Elderly patients, FDA tips for, 15

ENDIT trial, 119

Endpoints, 16, 18

Ephedra, 149

Erythromycin, 135, 180

Evening primrose oil, 74

# F

FDA
regulations, 8–10
tips, 14–16

Fenofibrate, 64

Fenugreek, 6, 66–68, 172

Feverfew interactions
garlic, 79
ginkgo, 84, 173
guggul, 97, 175
tea/caffeine, 150, 182

Fish oil, 69–73, 172

Fluconazole (Diflucan), 135, 149

Fluoroquinolones, 114, 149, 177

Fluoxetine (Prozac), 139

Fluvoxamine (Luvox), 136, 149

Fosamax, 114, 177

Fraud, spotting, 14–15

# G

Gamma-linolenic acid, 69, 74–76, 172

Gamma-tocopherol, 156

Garlic interactions
alcohol, 80, 173
fenugreek, 68
ginkgo, 84, 173
holy basil, 103, 176
overview, 77–80, 173
statin interactions, 97, 173
tea/caffeine, 150, 182

Gemfibrozil (Lopid), 136, 180

# L

Lactation. *See* Breast feeding drug interactions

L-carnitine, 65, 171

Lisinopril (Zestril), 163

Lithium, 149

Liver disease, 115–117, 148

Lopid, 160

Lovastatin (Mevacor), 130, 133, 180

Lovaza, 70, 71

# M

Magnesium, 110–114, 177

Metformin, 5, 35, 117, 168, 174

Miglitol (Glyset), 140

Milk thistle, 115–117, 178

Monacolins, 133

Monoamine oxidase (MAO) inhibitors, 149

# N

NATHAN I/II trials, 29

National Cholesterol Education Program (NCEP) Step-2 diet, 90–91

National Health and Nutrition Examination Survey, 156

Native Americans, 3

Natural Products Association, 12

Natural Standard, 13

Nefazodone (Serzone), 135–136

Nephropathy, 33

Neuropathy, 26, 33, 74–76

Niacin (vitamin B3), 136

Nicotinamide, 118–121, 178

Nicotine, 150

Night vision, 36–38

Nopal, 122–124

NSF International, 11

# O

Omega-3 plant oils, 69

Open-label studies, 18

Orlistat, 160, 183

Oxidative stress, 26

# P

Peanut allergy, 68

Penicillin, 174

Pentobarbital, 150

Pepcid, 55

Phenobarbital, 136, 160, 176, 183

Phenothiazines, 76

Phenylketonuria, 46

Phenytoin (Dilantin) interactions
red yeast rice, 136
tea/caffeine, 150, 182
thiamine, 35
zinc, 164, 184

Phosphatidylcholine, 116

Picolinate salt. *See* Chromium

Pine bark extract, 125–128, 179

Placebos, 17–18

Platelet activity, 38

Policosanol, 129–132, 179

Prandin, 100

Prednisone, 164, 184

Pregnancy, drug interactions
    aloe, 25, 167
    bitter melon, 39
    chromium, 52
    fenugreek, 68, 172
    fish oil/PCBs, 83
    ginseng, 87, 174
    guggul, 97, 185
    gymnema, 100, 175
    magnesium, 110
    stevia, 144
    tea, 147, 148, 182
    vanadium, 153

Prickly pear, 122–124

Prilosec, 55

Primidone, 121

Propranolol, 97

Proton pump inhibitors, 55

Psyllium (blonde), 43–46, 169

Pycnogenol, 125–128, 179

# R

Randomization, 17

Red yeast rice, 65, 133–136, 171, 180

Retinopathy, 33, 36, 37, 82, 126–127

Rhabdomyolysis, 135, 136, 180

Riboflavin, 46

Rosiglitazone (Avandia), 115

Run-in phase, 18

# S

Sábila. *See* Aloe vera

Salacia, 140–141, 181

Salba, 50–51

Secretagogues, 141, 150, 175, 176, 181

Seizures, 76, 83

Sertraline (Zoloft), 139

Side effects, 5–6, 15–16. *See also specific supplements*

Silymarin, 115–117

Simvastatin (Zocor), 115

Smoking, 64, 150

Snellen test, 127

Spironolactone, 114, 177

St. John's wort, 6, 136–139, 180

Starlix, 100

Statin interactions
    blonde psyllium, 169
    coenzyme Q10, 60–61, 64–65, 171
    garlic, 97, 173
    guggul, 175
    St. John's wort, 129–130, 139, 180
    vitamin E, 159, 183

Statistical significance, 19

Steroids, 111, 114, 128, 164, 170, 179, 184

Stevia, 142–145, 181

Study design, 17

Sudafed, 149

Sulfonylurea interactions. *See also* Glibenclamide; Glipizide; Glyburide
    aloe, 25, 167
    alpha-lipoic acid, 30, 167

# OTHER TITLES AVAILABLE FROM
# THE AMERICAN DIABETES ASSOCIATION

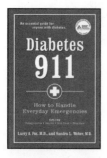

### Diabetes 911: How to Handle Everyday Emergencies
*by Larry A. Fox, MD, and Sandra L. Weber, MD*
When it comes to a condition as serious as diabetes, the best way to solve problems is to prevent them from ever happening. Do you know what to do in case of an emergency? With *Diabetes 911*, you will learn the necessary skills to handle hypoglycemia, insulin pump malfunctions, natural disasters, travel, depression, and sick days.
**Order no. 4887-01; Price $12.95**

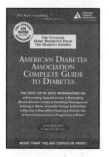

### American Diabetes Association
### Complete Guide to Diabetes, 4th Edition
*by American Diabetes Association*
Have all the tips and information on diabetes that you need close at hand. The world's largest collection of diabetes self-care tips, techniques, and tricks for solving diabetes-related problems is back in its fourth edition, and it's bigger and better than ever before.
**Order no. 4809-04; New low price $19.95**

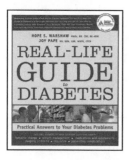

### Real-Life Guide to Diabetes
*by Hope S. Warshaw, MMSc, RD, CDE, BC-ADM, and Joy Pape, RN, BSC, CDE, WOCN, CFCN*
*Real-Life Guide* puts everything you need to know about diabetes into a one-of-a-kind book packed with the information you won't find anywhere else. Learn to prevent long-term complications, understand the ins and outs of health insurance, work physical activity into your daily life, and control your blood glucose, cholesterol, and blood pressure. Bring a realistic approach to your diabetes care plan.
**Order no. 4893-01; Price $19.95**

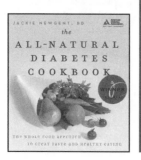

### The All-Natural Diabetes Cookbook:
### The Whole Food Approach to Great Taste and Healthy Eating
*by Jackie Newgent, RD*
Instead of relying on artificial sweeteners or not-so-real substitutions to reduce calories, sugar, and fat, *The All-Natural Diabetes Cookbook* takes a different approach, focusing on naturally delicious fresh foods and whole-food ingredients to create fantastic meals that deliver amazing taste and well-rounded nutrition. And absolutely nothing is artificial.
**Order no. 4663-01; Price $18.95**

To order these and other great American Diabetes Association titles,
call 1-800-232-6733 or visit http://store.diabetes.org.
American Diabetes Association titles are also available in bookstores nationwide.